Advance Care Planning

Prepare for Serious Illness by Sharing Your Wishes for Future Health and Personal Care

Connie Jorsvik, BSN

Self-Counsel Press
(a division of)
International Self-Counsel Press Ltd.
Canada   USA

Self-Counsel Press acknowledges the financial support of the Government of Canada through the Canada Book Fund (CBF) for our publishing activities.

Printed in Canada.   Canadä

First edition: 2020

Library and Archives Canada Cataloguing in Publication

Title: Advance care planning : prepare for serious illness by sharing your wishes for future health and personal care / Connie Jorsvik.

Names: Jorsvik, Connie, author.

Series: Healthcare series (Self-Counsel Press)

Description: First edition. | Series statement: Healthcare series

Identifiers: Canadiana (print) 2020019772X | Canadiana (ebook) 20200197878 | ISBN 9781770403253 (softcover) | ISBN 9781770405103 (EPUB) | ISBN 9781770405110 (Kindle)

Subjects: LCSH: Advance directives (Medical care)—Popular works. | LCSH: Older people—Medical care—Popular works. | LCSH: Older people—Life skills guides. | LCSH: Wills—Popular works. | LCSH: Estate planning—Popular works.

Classification: LCC R726.2 .J67 2020 | DDC 646.7/9—dc23

Excerpts from the following used with permission:

Dying with Dignity Canada

Kenneth Rockwood, MD: Clinical Frailty Index

Every effort has been made to obtain permission for quoted material and illustrations. If there is an omission or error, the author and publisher would be grateful to be so informed.

Self-Counsel Press
(a division of)
International Self-Counsel Press Ltd.

North Vancouver, BC   Bellingham, WA
Canada   USA

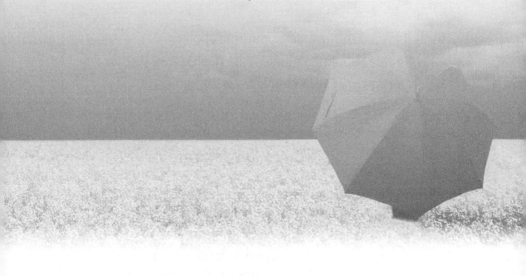

Contents

CHAPTER FOUR: In Case of Emergency (ICE):
A Form That Communicates When You Can't

CHAPTER FIVE: Financial Planning for Serious Illness,
Injury, and Disability

Notice to Readers

Laws are constantly changing. Every effort is made to keep this publication as current as possible. However, the author, the publisher, and the vendor of this book make no representations or warranties regarding the outcome or the use to which the information in this book is put and are not assuming any liability for any claims, losses, or damages arising out of the use of this book. The reader should not rely on the author or the publisher of this book for any professional advice. Please be sure that you have the most recent edition.

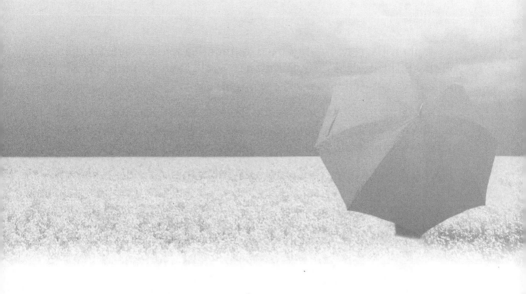

Acknowledgements

I want to thank my team at Patient Pathways for their hard work and cheerleading: Kerry Phillips, Vicki Lee, and my team of navigator advocates. We are changing the health-care system!

To the growing number of women and men who have started their own end-of-life businesses and are changing the way we see and approach our inevitable ending. You are a constant inspiration to me. I am so proud to call you friends:

Dr. Sue Hughson, who brought me into this incredible tribe. You continue to be a beacon for patient choice.

Michelle and Reena at Willow End of Life who are bringing joy to the process through their programs, tools, and workshops on the opportunities of mortality; leaving a legacy and heart letters; and decisions on how people want to leave this life.

Ngaio Davis, at KORU Cremation and Burial, who has brought beauty, love, and light back into the end of people's lives. There are no somber funeral parlours here. She is pushing boundaries and is always a resource for me and for my clients.

Stephen Garrett, Death Coach, author, leader, teacher. Stephen, your no-BS attitude is an inspiration to us all. I love hanging out with you and wish we could do it more often.

Dr. Marylene Kyriazus, Frankie Hester, and Dr. Paul Sugar of the Paul Sugar Palliative Support Centre in North Vancouver, who have taught me, supported my journey, and loved me.

And, to the entire team at Dying with Dignity Canada, especially Alex Muir, Susan Jobes, and Maureen Aslin, and the team of volunteers in Vancouver and across the country I am honoured to work beside. I have never met and worked with such incredible, passionate people. You are helping to change the landscape of dying in Canada.

Introduction:
Advance Care Planning

This book is for every person, at any age, and stage of life and health. It is about taking back control of your body and your health decisions; learning how to better communicate with your health-care teams; and while important and often ignored, planning for serious illness and, eventually, for the end of your life.

The concepts of "patient-centered care" and "shared decision making" have been a part of medical theory for at least 30 years but in our fast-paced, overburdened health-care system, the person who is patient gets left behind. This is a basic guide that will help you be a part of your own care and decision making so that you are hopefully not one of the unfortunate ones left behind.

As a health-care navigator and patient advocate, my clients are often in crisis. I have tried to summarize and give all patients and families the same advice I would as if I were in the room with them.

When you are seriously ill and your health-care team is not listening to you, or have told you what you are experiencing is "all in your head, " this book may help, but you will likely need advice that is beyond what is offered here. I will give you some ideas in Chapter 1 on how to find resources that might help.

Part 1 of this book is about the basics of patient and caregiver empowerment. Part 2 is a deep-dive into planning for serious injury, illness, or end of life — whether you're still healthy, facing illness and frailty, or in the midst of a health crisis that is life-threatening.

As we begin to look at becoming empowered, it's interesting to look back and see the road of the empowered patient.

The empowered patient movement began in earnest in the 1960s and 1970s when women started to have a choice about their bodies and control of their lives. First came the birth control pill, and suddenly women had a choice over when, if, and how many children they would have. Birth rates plummeted in the Western world and as that happened, women slowly began to move into male-dominated careers, including medicine.

In 1979, I was a senior nursing student in Victoria, BC, doing one of my rotations in maternity. A massive change — almost an earthquake — was taking place at that very moment. In nursing classes, we were learning about Lamaze and other natural birthing methods, and that women were pushing to go back to using midwives and having home births. As students, we had vigorous debates over rights and choice versus the safety of mothers and babies.

And then we stepped into the real world of antiquated deliveries and I could see why mothers wanted to go back to delivering in their own homes and beds. Birthing was a cold, sterile, and uncomfortable experience. I remember everything being white, from the walls to the bedding. The beds were uncomfortable and there were no options for a more comfortable labour: there were no baths, no showers, and no other labour assistance tools. Women were behind closed doors, without spouses or birth coaches, and were encouraged to "labour quietly." When they were finally ready to push, we ran for a stretcher and between heavy contractions would whip the mother onto the stretcher and down the hall to the sterile birthing room and place her on a medieval contraption that was no different than a gynecologist's table with stirrups. She would push, with her feet in the horrible contraptions until she delivered — sometimes two or three hours later.

The maternity ward was another regimented unit, where babies were bundled tightly, put on a cart like a bunch of adorable sausages, and delivered to their mothers every four hours. They were left for 30 minutes to feed and cuddle, and then bundled back up and taken back to the nursery. If babies needed to be fed in between, we gave them sugar water or formula. New moms were in hospital for four to six days.

I had just gotten married and was thinking about having babies, but I knew I didn't want to have them like that. It turned out a lot of other women didn't want it either. Within four years, every maternity ward and hospital began to change. Beautiful and comfortable birthing suites became the norm and rooming-in with babies became standard. Within seven years, most new moms and their babies were going home within 24 hours.

While the old guard of nurses and doctors did not go willingly or happily into the good night, it was a mother-driven uprising.

Now, this same group of adults is changing the way we want health care delivered and how we want the end of our lives to look. We keep pushing for choice and we're not prepared to stop.

It shouldn't be surprising that almost all those who attend my Empowered Patient and Advance Care Planning workshops are women. They have been the mothers and the caregivers and they have seen what happens when we don't plan.

Women are still not being taken as seriously as men when we are sick. It is much more likely that our symptoms will be dismissed or that we will receive a psychiatric diagnosis. It is a theme that has gone back centuries. Through social media, women are fighting back. An example is an incredible video, produced in BC and viewed, as of this writing, almost 18 million times in 190 countries. It is *A Typical Heart* (Distillery Film Company, 2019), about the underdiagnosis and undertreatment of women and heart disease — the leading cause of death in women currently. It will change the way women are treated in cardiac care.

In Canada, we are at the forefront in change for choice at the end of our lives. Medical Assistance in Dying (MAiD) began as a grass-roots movement with Sue Rodriguez asking for the right to assisted death in 1993 (Assisted Suicide in Canada: The Rodriguez Case [1993]: www.thecanadianencyclopedia.ca/en/article/rodriguez-case-1993). It's been a legal choice since 2016 and that choice is changing everything. We want to get all the care and treatment Western medicine can offer us, but then we can choose to say, "That's enough. I'm ready to die."

Informed and responsible choices along our health-care journeys are the basis of being empowered patients and caregivers. We need to assertively ask for a seat at our own health-care discussions and decisions.

"What you feel is real and important and you should never feel afraid to communicate that." (Dr. Doreen Rabi, Clinical Endocrinologist, University of Calgary — in *A Typical Heart*.)

For many of us, the thought of being in a care facility for severe disability or advanced dementia is untenable. Advance care planning, detailed advance directives, and the option of MAiD, gives us options as far as how we choose the ends of our lives to look.

Our society is in a health-care crisis. There are not enough hospital beds, nurses, doctors, or allied health professionals. But there is an antidote: Educate yourself; be an active participant in your own care; be responsible for your own body and mind; and be respectful as you communicate, plan ahead through advance care planning conversations, and document and proactively communicate with all involved in your care.

1. How This Book Works

The first step in working this book to ensure your rights and desires are taken care of is to know your patient rights. While each province has developed its own health care legislation to be discussed throughout the book, there is a national framework in Canada that, when broken down, ensures very CAPABLE adult has the right to —

- be fully informed of all treatment options,

- have his or her Substitute Decision Maker recognized,

- have his or her Advance Directive (a document that can go by other names as well, see Chapter 8) followed,

- pain and symptom management,

- refuse treatment,

- end his or her own life, and

- assisted death.

There are two parts to the book. Part 1 is about the basics of empowerment and navigating the health-care system. Part 2 is about determining what your wishes are and deciding how best to communicate them to loved ones and health-care providers.

There is also a downloadable forms kit included with more resources for you to use (see URL at the back of this book to access it).

Communication and preparation are the two biggest keys to successfully navigating our complex health-care system. The work required of readers in the upcoming chapters is not easy, but it's incredibly rewarding to come out the other end with a lot of knowledge and a plan.

PART
ONE

Empowered Patients and Caregivers: Navigating the Canadian Health-Care System

In this first part of the book, we will discuss how to –

- be an active participant in your own or your loved one's health care,

- improve communication at all points in the health-care journey,

- effectively navigate the health-care system,

- prepare for medical emergencies, and

- prepare financially for serious illness, injury, and disability.

CHAPTER
ONE

Become an Empowered Patient or Caregiver

Each of us has multiple names for the roles we have in our lives: mother, father, sister, brother, daughter, son, boss, employee, coach, or volunteer. However, unless we are on our way to a health appointment with our doctor, our physiotherapist, registered massage therapist, etc., or in an emergency room or in hospital, we rarely think of ourselves as a patient.

Almost everyone has been a patient and will likely be one in the future. It is something you can prepare for to some degree. It can be the most complex role of your life.

We don't have crystal balls — and that's likely a good thing — but chances are high each one of us will be significantly impacted by serious injury or complex illness, either because we are injured or ill ourselves, or because an injury or illness is affecting someone we love. And, most of us have been or will be a caregiver.

This book is about how to become more empowered and more prepared. When we are empowered, we educate ourselves, we speak up, and we are active participants in our own and our loved ones' health care.

Becoming empowered — being an active participant in your own health care — is borne out of necessity. We must learn these skills on the fly when we are thrown into a world few of us understand. Being an empowered patient means being responsible, diligent, open to learning, questioning, and trying to be prepared. However, none of us can be empowered all the time. You simply can't fully be prepared for injury and illness, but thinking about it before it happens will go a long way to successfully navigating the complicated health-care system.

As an empowered patient:

- You understand your rights as patient and those of any substitute decision makers.

- You are in charge of your body, mind, and spirit.

- You actively learn about your health and understand your health conditions.

- It's your life and your choice how to live it — including how to spend the end of your life.

- You collaborate with your health-care team to make a decision that is right for you and, as a result, are more likely to follow through on care and treatments.

- You want to be treated as a person and not as a patient.

- You think about what you want for your life when you are seriously ill or injured and make your family and future decision makers aware of your wishes.

- You are better prepared to talk with your health-care provider.

The opposite of empowered means giving your power away

Margaret was 69 years old. I was her preoperative nurse and had been admitting her for a relatively minor surgery.

"Have you had surgery in the past?" I asked.

"Yes, a couple of times, a few years ago," she replied.

Most people have a pretty good understanding of any surgeries they've had in their adult years, even if the dates are murky, but Margaret couldn't give me any details. I did a head-to-toe exam and found two significant incisional scars on her abdomen that could have been either from a C-section or hysterectomy, and something that looked like it might have been from having her gallbladder removed. More prodding into her history revealed she had never had children, so a C-section was off the list, meaning the lower scar was likely from a hysterectomy. I was perplexed. "You don't have any idea what this surgery was for?" She was as frustrated as I was. "Look, if my doctor tells me I need surgery, I have the surgery. I don't want to know why, and I don't want to know the details. And, I don't want to know what this surgery is about either, so you can leave your teaching and your pamphlets for someone else!"

Margaret was the opposite of an empowered patient. Some people simply don't want to be involved in their own care, they have no understanding of their body, and they leave everything, good and bad, to their doctors and nurses. It can be a very dangerous and deadly attitude.

---

1. Becoming and Remaining an Empowered Patient

When you are seriously ill or injured — and most certainly when you're diagnosed with a neurological injury/disease or you have had a diagnosis of dementia — the last thing you will want to do is stand up for yourself. But, being seriously injured or ill isn't like having a bad cold or flu, where being empowered is a sprint. This will be a marathon.

I have heard the same line from dozens of people: "I'm done. I'm just done." They're out of fight and out of reserves. They want to hand this over to a navigator like me or to their loved ones. We can take some of it on, but we can't take on the aches, the pains, the brain fog, and we can't go to doctor's appointments, treatments, or surgeries.

It is hard, and ultimately, lonely work. You must stay organized. This is a big job; maybe, the biggest of your life. You are a patient because this requires patience and persistence; sometimes far beyond your limits. But, there really isn't any choice. There is no magic pill (except for opioids that have their own dire, life-threatening consequences) to make things all better. You must keep standing up for yourself and ask for the information and help that you need.

Seek all the support you can possibly find. Find a therapist (as easy as a Google search for your area) who is trained in helping people with chronic illness, injury, and pain. Take care of yourself: Do everything you can to take in a healthy diet; sleep eight to nine hours a night; push yourself to remain active, and exercise as much as you can.

Look for minor gains and build on those. Write a journal to look back on your progress.

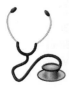

Practice gratitude. "The things we love won't cure our illnesses. There still will be medications with rotten side effects and symptoms that make us feel lousy. But they can make our illnesses easier to bear. Even on horrible days when pain is unrelenting and hope is dim, these "good things" we carry within us sustain us by reminding us that we are more than our suffering." ("Cultivating Gratitude while Living with Chronic Illness," PsychologyToday.com, accessed January, 2020.)

Being grateful doesn't mean you won't feel pain and grief, but it can make feelings more bearable and even reduce depression.

1.1 Build your team

1.1a Get your doctors on side

The health-care system is not always on board with us being a part of our own team. Doctors often don't talk to each other, let alone their patients. They often only have time to have a cursory read of your chart, write a few orders, and move on. It's important for you to have assertive discussions with your doctors and let them know that is your expectation to be fully informed and part of your health care.

If you are an empowered patient in the community, do your homework on picking your doctors. Switching general practitioners (GPs) can be a challenge, particularly in rural areas where choice may be limited.

It's important to find a doctor who will listen and treat you as an intelligent, well-informed patient. If you are being referred to a specialist, do the homework for your doctor and provide a short-list of specialists who are best suited for your needs and have good WebMD ratings. (See Chapter 3 for more.)

Remaining an empowered patient or caregiver in the hospital is more difficult because you can't choose any of your health-care team.

You will need knowledge and assertiveness, mixed with a healthy dose of empathy for health-care constraints, kindness, and gratitude (when earned), to help you get the health care you need and deserve.

1.2 The power of empowered caregivers

Through planning and having vital discussions prior to serious injury or illness, an empowered caregiver can step in when you are seriously ill, injured, or your ability to think and plan is reduced due to medications (especially narcotics), head injuries, dementia, or serious mental health issues.

In Canada, the person helping you to make your decisions is called your Substitute Decision Maker (SDM). (Your SDM can be formalized in a legal document that we'll go over later on in this book.) Every province has its own legislation and required documents and those will be outlined in the Resources section at the end of this book. There are ways you can make it easier for your SDM to get information on your behalf and help you make decisions.

In hospital, doctors are always in a hurry and it's hard for them to plan to meet with or call loved ones and SDMs. Doctors' rounds are often very early in the morning, and after their office hours or surgeries are completed; it is often up to your SDM to be with you when the doctor is most likely to arrive. This can mean early mornings and long days waiting for your doctor. That waiting for care is literally the meaning of being "patient."

Becoming a caregiver is rarely something we plan for. In case of a serious injury or illness of a loved one, the need to step into this role can be sudden and overwhelming. One minute you are leading your own life and the next you are submersed in the health-care system, learning the medical language and routines, spending significant time in the hospital at your loved one's side. You will likely have to take time off work and your own commitments. You may need to leave your own home and find accommodation close to the hospital. And, the financial expenses and loss of income can be overwhelming.

You will likely need to step into the role of nurse and caregiver when your loved one comes home, often long before you feel they are ready. You may need to coordinate home care, rehabilitation, and physician appointments. This can last for weeks, months, or years.

Case Study

As an empowered caregiver you often put your own life on hold.

Even those who have a health-care background can struggle when advocating for themselves or others. Maggie had been an RN for 30 years when her son, Jack, 22, had a serious, life-threatening head and neck injury. He was in the ICU for almost two months and then in rehabilitation for another six months. He struggled physically and psychologically for another two years.

Maggie was forced to take time off from work for several months and life didn't return to normal for years. She was Jack's advocate from the moment she saw him in ICU on a ventilator, through countless specialist appointments, and then to psychiatrists' offices as he struggled through significant depression and Intensive Care Unit (ICU) induced PTSD.

"Being a nurse, I thought I'd be better prepared," she said. "It's different when you're up over your head in this system and it's someone you love." It took a long time for her to put away the notebooks and diaries, textbooks, and medical articles that had built up on her dining room table.

Jack's story has a happy ending. He went back to university and now has a job that he loves. He never hesitates to give his mom the credit she deserves for being his advocate, and on several occasions, for undoubtedly saving his life.

2. Becoming a Caregiver after Serious Injury and During Illness

When you or a loved one is seriously ill or injured, you will find yourself pushed into the deep end of the health-care system. Knowing who is who in the zoo and what their role is will help you to survive and thrive.

As quickly as possible, find out who the key health-care professionals are on the hospital unit where your loved one is receiving care.

Find out who the nurse who runs the unit on a day-to-day basis: The name is different in just about every hospital and every unit (examples: head nurse, patient-care coordinator, nurse manager). This nurse is usually there for several shifts in a row and has ongoing knowledge of all the patients and what the nurses, doctors, physiotherapists, and occupational therapists are saying and doing. Introduce yourself and ask for an introduction as to the layout of the unit, phone numbers, best times to call, and when doctors are most likely to make rounds. Write this all in your notebook.

2.1 Who is who

- **Registered Nurses (RN):** They are often key allies in getting information and keeping you in the loop. Write down their names and the dates and times of the shifts they worked (in case something goes wrong — but, also, if you later want to send a thank you).

- **Unit social worker (SW):** Can be a key resource for all things non-medical such as emergency financial resources, psychological supports, and are often a key-player in planning for discharge or transfer to other units, services, and home.

- **Physiotherapists (PT):** The key persons in getting patients physically activated, transferring from bed to chair and toilet, walking, and strong enough to get home. Ask to be taught how to help with physical exercises.

- **Occupational Therapists (OT):** They help with assessment of how a patient can do their activities of daily living (eating, bathing, dressing, toileting, and self-care). The OT will be responsible for assessments for where your loved one will go next: rehabilitation, residential care, or home. They are key players in discharge planning and any equipment that will be needed if the patient is going home.

- **Physicians:** These are the key-players you are likely to see the least. Who the doctors are, depends on the unit the patient is on, and the size of the hospital. If the patient is in a smaller hospital, the family physician will likely remain involved and be the lead physician. In larger hospitals, on general nursing units, **hospitalists** (who are general practitioners or internal medicine specialists) are assigned to be the lead in patient teams. They usually will have rotations of a week or two, so there is consistent medical care. In critical care and intensive care units, specialists will likely lead the teams and are on-duty or available 24 hours a day. In large teaching hospitals you may never see the lead physicians and specialists, as all care will be overseen by Residents. Wherever possible, ask questions of who the doctors are and try to get an understanding of their rotations and availability.

- **Most Responsible Physician/Practitioner (MRP)**: This is the physician or nurse practitioner who is ultimately responsible for the patient's care. This role is most often used in larger hospitals, and when multiple specialists are involved in care, and the role is often assigned according to the primary reason the patient was admitted to hospital (cardiology, neurology, orthopedics, internal medicine). Sometimes, the MRP gets lost in the shuffle, especially when the patient is moved from a critical care unit to a nursing unit. This can result in a lack of oversight and planning. It is vital to know who your MRP is and to make sure they continue to oversee the patient's care.

2.2 Caregiving when loved ones have chronic illness and increasing frailty

As we age, chronic conditions begin to multiply and our need for assistance begins slowly: grocery shopping, assistance to get to and from an increasing number of doctors' appointments, help with housekeeping, meal preparation, and help with medications. Most of us — 70 to 80 percent of us, will rely on family caregivers after serious illness or increasing frailty. In fact, our health-care system demands that family caregivers be involved, even after serious health setbacks such as hip repairs, strokes, and increasing dementia. There are long wait lists for assisted living and long-term care beds in every community across the country, and only those with advanced dementia or complete disability even qualify for the wait lists. It can be a very long, underappreciated, underpaid role.

The average age for adult children caring for their aging parents is 45 to 65, often at the height of their own careers. The burden of multiple roles can be overwhelming. The slide into the caregiving role is often subtle with a few errands here or there, sometimes rising sharply as a result of a serious fall, unsafe behaviours such as wandering or leaving appliances on, or an admission to hospital with an escalation of a preexisting condition.

When you find yourself caring for a loved one, seek information and resources early. Call your local community health centre and ask to speak to a case manager or social worker. Seek information on how to take care of yourself so you can better care for those you love.

Because of our rapidly aging population, there is an ever-growing number of adult children who are retired but still looking after very aged parents.

Case Study

Lisa was 70 and her mother 95 years old when she began reaching out to as many professionals as she could find to help her with the increasingly challenging task of safely keeping her mother at home as long as possible while planning ahead for long-term care.

Her mother, Betty, had limited financial resources and private home care or residential care were not options. Lisa did the best she could with the government resources provided. She communicated regularly with her mother's home-health case manager to maximize publicly subsidized companion care to help with bathing, dressing, and light meal preparation. That still left a lot of gaps in her mother's needs and she reached out to community organizations for volunteers to take her mother out for walks and activities.

Despite all the care that was being provided by others, Lisa needed to coordinate care and attend increasing numbers of doctor's appointments. She was becoming mentally exhausted and saw the signs of caregiver burnout happening: She was increasingly short-tempered, impatient, and emotionally and physically fatigued.

She reached out to a therapist who counselled family caregivers. She found the support she needed to set boundaries, find additional resources to allow her more time for herself, and let go of the guilt and resentment that had built up.

Her mother died relatively suddenly and peacefully several months later. The work that Lisa had done for her self-care meant that her grief was relatively uncomplicated. Lisa misses her mom, but the negative emotions of guilt and resentment were minimal.

3. When You Need to Hire a Professional Navigator-Advocate

Independent patient navigation and advocacy is starting to grow as a profession in Canada. Navigator-advocates play a vital role for

Table 1
Health Information Resources by Province

Province	Community Referrals and Information	Services	Health-Care Referrals and Information	Services
British Columbia	**BC 211** www.bc211.ca Call or text: 2-1-1	Provides information and referral regarding community, government, and social services in BC. The help line services include 211, the Alcohol and Drug Information and Referral Service (ADIRS), the Gambling Support Line BC, the Shelter and Street Help Line, VictimLink BC, and the Youth Against Violence Line.	**Healthlink BC** www.healthlinkbc.ca Call 8-1-1, 24/7	Health service navigators help you find information or health services, or connect you with a nurse or dietician.
Alberta	**211 Alberta** www.ab.211.ca Call or text: 2-1-1	A helpline and website that provides information on and referrals to Alberta's community, social, health-related and government services.	**811 Health Link** www.albertahealth services.ca/assets/healthinfo/link/index.html Call 8-1-1, 24/7	Provides clinical services including tele-triage and health advice, navigation services, and online content support.
Saskatchewan	**211 Saskatchewan** sk.211.ca/homepage Call or text: 2-1-1	Free, confidential, 24/7 service that connects individuals to human services in the province by telephone, text, or web chat, plus a searchable website with over 5,000 listings of social, community, non-clinical health, and government services across the province.	**Healthline 811** www.saskatchewan.ca/residents/health/accessing-health-care-services/healthline Call 8-1-1, 24/7	Confidential, 24-hour health and mental health and addictions advice, education, and support. It is staffed by Registered Nurses, Registered Psychiatric Nurses, and Registered Social Workers.
Manitoba	**211 Manitoba** mb.211.ca Call: 2-1-1	Searchable online database of government, health, and social services across the province. Services are grouped together into categories that include food and clothing, housing, and homelessness, health, mental health, employment, newcomers, children and parenting, and youth.	**MBTelehealth** mbtelehealth.ca 1-866-999-9696 (Option 4)	Access to health services through the use of technologies, to overcome the barriers of distance, time, and expense, and provides tools that connect people to the information and services they require to manage their health and well-being closer to home.

Table 1 – Continued

Province	Community Referrals and Information	Services	Health-Care Referrals and Information	Services
Ontario	**211 Ontario** https://211ontario.ca Call: 2-1-1 Email and live chat from website.	Connects people to the right information and health and human services.	**OTN.ca (Ontario Telehealth)** https://otn.ca **eMentalHealth.ca** https://www.ementalhealth.ca/Ontario/Home/index.php?m=home 1-866-797-0000	By maximizing access to care and minimizing travel and wait times, virtual care makes health care delivery more human, efficient, and equitable. Free, confidential telephone service to get health advice or general health information from a Registered Nurse 24/7.
New Brunswick	**211 New Brunswick** http://www.nbinfo.ca Call: 2-1-1	Provides online information regarding community services including health, social, and government services	**Tele-care 811** https://www2.gnb.ca/content/gnb/en/departments/health/Tele-Care.html Call: 8-1-1, 24/7	Free, confidential, health advice and information line.
Newfoundland and Labrador	No local partner		**NL Healthline** Dept of Health & Community Services **CALL 811 or Tel:** 1-888-709-2929 **TTY:** 1-888-709-3555	Trained nurses help you decide what steps to manage your physical and mental health, and provide health services information.
Nova Scotia	**211 Nova Scotia** http://ns.211.ca/ Call: 2-1-1	Free, confidential information and referral service that can connect you to thousands of programs and services offered by local community groups, nonprofits, and government departments.	**811 Healthline** https://www.811healthline.ca Call 8-1-1, 24/7 or 1-888-709-2929	Trained nurses help you decide what steps to manage your physical and mental health, 211, and provide health services information.
Prince Edward Island	As of the time of writing, 211PEI is being built and will be launched by Spring 2020.	Free confidential information and referral service to community, social, and government services 24/7 by phone or online database.	**811 Telehealth** https://www.princeedwardisland.ca/en/information/health-and-wellness/811-telehealth Call: 8-1-1, 24/7	A registered nurse is available 24 hours a day to answer your health questions over the phone and will help you determine whether you require emergency or non-urgent medical attention; provide current, reliable information related to your health issue; and offer helpful guidance about health services.

Table 1 – Continued

Province	Community Referrals and Information	Services	Health-Care Referrals and Information	Services
Nunavut	www/nu.211.ca	Provides reliable information about the program and services available.	No local partner	
Northwest Territories	No local partner		No local partner	
Yukon	No local partner		**Healthline 811** http://www.hss. gov.yk.ca/811. php Call: 8-1-1 or by satellite phone to 1-604-215-4700 (Healthlink BC)	Health and social services: Staffed by registered nurses who can answer your health questions or direct you to someone in your community who can assist you.

patients and families who are separated by geographical distances, work and family commitments, or who are overwhelmed by a process they don't understand. Navigator-advocates can be worth every penny because they are working for the patient and the family, and not the government or the health-care system. They are your voice and they understand the system.

Definitions of roles:

- Navigators walk with you in your health-care journey. It is a supportive role and a navigator is a member of your team. Health-care professionals generally recognize the support navigators provide and welcome them to your consultations and appointments.

- Advocates walk ahead of you. They lead the way rather than merely being at your side. There are times, such as when registering a complaint, that this becomes necessary. They strive to be nonconfrontational and to promote dialogue.

If you are going to hire a navigator-advocate, do your homework:

- What experience does the person have that is relevant to your situation?

- What education does the person bring? If he or she is not a health-care professional by training, what other education does he or she have that is relevant?

Find navigator-advocates in your area by doing web searches with the key word searches: [name of city and province] + health care + patient + navigator + advocate.

Find Canadian navigator-advocates that are with the US-based organization APHA (Alliance of Professional Health Advocates). These navigator-advocates must meet minimum standards to be a part of the organization: https://aphadvocates.org/directory.

Like all health-care professionals, references can be hard to come by, as most clients want to remain anonymous. Read the "About Us" biographies; be sure to look for testimonials on websites; and be prepared to ask the navigator questions about how long they've been in health care and their level of expertise.

4. Empowered Patients and Caregivers (a Review)

- As a patient or caregiver, ask for help when you need it. No one should be in our complex, fragmented health-care system alone.

- Get your doctors and health-care team on side: Be assertive, be responsible, gather your own information, and share your questions and concerns.

- If you are alone or separated by time or distance from your support system, hire a professional navigator-advocate, if possible, before you're in crisis.

- Get supports in place so that you can stay empowered over the long term.

CHAPTER
TWO
Empowered Communication

Communication is at the heart of being an empowered, an informed, and a responsible patient and caregiver. It is the most important, vital, and highly underrated tool in your health-care toolbox. If you are in a health crisis, this is a crash course.

Our complex, siloed, fragmented health care works because of the incredible dedication of the people who go above and beyond, every single day. Our health-care system is organized chaos, dependent on tens of thousands of doctors, nurses, allied professionals, and support staff who are often unsung heroes.

In health care, every person on your team is equally responsible for doing each step right. When things go wrong, it is nearly always a result of a communication failure. Successful communication starts with the patient, and the patient's back-up team of loved ones, caregivers, and substitute decision makers.

When I act as a health-care navigator and patient advocate, the only tool I have is to listen and then begin to repair communication holes and fractures. I help patients clarify their health and treatment priorities; I push doctors to talk to patients and families; I help teams plan for effective and safe discharge home; help families talk to frazzled community case managers; and work with fractured families so the patient is the number one concern. With a little practice and coaching, everyone can do the same.

1. No One Should Be Alone in the Health-Care System

Our health-care professionals are human and they make mistakes. Often, communication between staff is missed due to overwhelming workloads. But, nearly everyone in the health-care system is trying his or her best. The problem is generally not them — it is that our system is highly complex.

I still have my old textbooks from nursing school. The information and pictures in them are almost laughable in their simplicity. When I graduated, our hospital in Victoria in 1980, BC boasted having the first CT scanner on Vancouver Island. Within months, the wait time to get a scan was several months. Now, every major hospital has two or three CT scanners, an MRI machine, and often a PET scanner. Laboratory technology has also exploded in growth. Yet we can't keep up with the demand.

People are no sicker than they were 50 years ago, we just have more tools to find a diagnosis and more ways to fix — and a much bigger population that is rapidly aging. People used to just die but now we try to fix everything, no matter how old we are. The tenth edition of the World Health Organization international classification of diseases now has listed more than 13,000 different diseases, syndromes, and types of injury (International Statistical Classification of Disease and Health Related Problems: The ICD-10, Second Edition: apps.who.int/bookorders/anglais/detart1.jsp?sesslan=1&codl an=1&codcol=15&codcch=1592).

Doctors, nurses, and other allied health professionals such as occupational therapists and physiotherapists, rarely have the time and resources to do their jobs the way they want or need. Communication can be ineffective within health-care teams — and major cracks and holes show up as you seek help for your serious personal health issues. It's why you need to be empowered and have people on your own personal team (or why you might want to be on a loved one's team) to watch, listen, and record.

2. The Power of a Notebook

A notebook is an essential tool of the empowered patient and his or her caregiver.

As a navigator-advocate, my notebook is my primary tool and I have taught dozens of patients and caregivers how to use it effectively. Consistent note taking improves communication, reduces errors, increases compliance, and helps save lives.

When there is a lot of information coming at you during an information-dense appointment, you retain as little as 7 to 17 percent of what is told to you within ten minutes. For example, a newly diagnosed cancer patient may see as many as 5 health-care professionals on a first visit, and 90 to 150 doctors over the course of treatment. No one can remember all the information — let alone when shocked, scared, and overwhelmed.

In these complex appointments, no matter our age and thinking ability, we must have someone with us to take notes. If a loved one is frail, due to health and/or age, it increases the importance of having someone with them to raise concerns and take vital and thorough notes at all appointments, even with the family doctor.

3. The Power of Being Respectfully Assertive

In order to get the best possible care, good communication skills become essential. Health-care professionals are under tremendous time pressure and there are more and more patients who are verbally and physically abusive toward them. Being respectful and understanding will earn good will and cooperation. Losing your temper or being disrespectful is likely to result in you being refused care. An assertive, kind, and respectful attitude always works better than aggressive, rude, or sarcastic behaviour.

4. The Power of Staying Logical in Doctors' Appointments

Staying calm, cool, and collected during doctor's appointments and health-care meetings can be an incredible challenge when you're scared, overwhelmed, or you aren't feeling heard and understood. Being overly emotional during health-care appointments can reduce doctor interaction and optimal care. Emotions can shut down conversations and you run the risk of being labelled with a somatization disorder (it's all in your head) or psychiatric condition. At worst, it will get you fired as a patient.

Navigator-advocates are often hired because patients are feeling unheard or even ignored. After a short evaluation, I often see that a patient has ineffective communication skills or habits. Some have cried through the consultation or slouched down in the chair so low as to be invisible. Many clients have said, "He needs to see how frustrated and angry I am! I'm just done!" Or, they're in a negative emotional state before going to see a new physician, "They all treat me like crap and have all of my life. All doctors are the same and this one isn't going to be any different!" and then go into the appointment angry and unwilling to take in any new information, and are much more likely to be uncompliant to proposed treatments.

Being overly emotional means that you are less likely to hear what your doctor has to say and interferes with information processing. When you are upset, the doctor will need to support your emotional well-being before getting relevant information from you and providing you with treatment advice.

Honey works so much better than vinegar. Be kind, leave your anger and frustration at the door, and show your doctor and nurses that you know they are busy and you appreciate their time.

- Write down what you need to accomplish in the appointment. If you are too upset to talk, hand the written list over to your doctor to read.

- Bring someone with you who can be calm, cool, and collected and have them take notes.

- See if you can visualize a "logic switch" and turn it on just long enough to get through the appointment.

- Be "in the moment": Listen and don't move onto your next thought or retort before the doctor is finished. Do positive self-talk immediately before the appointment: "I am calm and I am listening."

- Be clinical about your feelings when you are describing them to your doctors. "I am very nervous about this; this scares me; I am worried," and say those things as if you are someone else describing your emotions.

- Be aware of your body language: Sit up straight, arms softly at your sides, and look your doctor in the eyes.

- Avoid "but." "That's great but I've tried that before and it didn't work." It means you are not in full listening mode and "but" shuts down the conversation.

- Avoid applying an emotional context to the appointment: "He didn't like me; she is so arrogant; he'd already made up his mind; she wasn't taking me seriously." Doctors are often in a rush, in a hurry, logical, and are trained not to show excessive concern. How they react to you often has nothing to do with you.

- Never cry crocodile tears just to get a reaction. Doctors can see through fake emotions faster than the time it takes for you to sit down. Fake emotions are a sign of immaturity, lack of self-control, and manipulation.

All of this takes practice. If you've got a friend who's willing to do some play-acting with constructive feedback, give that a try. Better communication means better health care.

5. Effective Communication in Hospital Saves Lives

Every patient admitted to hospital — especially those older than the age of 65 — needs someone attentive to watch, listen, ask questions, and give reminders to the team about the patient's specific needs and concerns.

Having someone sitting beside you, holding your hand, is not enough. Your "person" needs to be responsible for asking questions. He or she is the one with the notebook who can write down the answers to questions such as:

1. Who came to see you?

   - Write the date and the name of your nurse, every shift. If everything goes well, you will have their names for a thank-you card, but if there are concerns in the future, you have this important information.

   - Who were the doctors who came to see you? Don't hesitate to ask two or three times who the doctors are and what their role is; they don't take offense. In big teaching hospitals, the turnover of hospitalists, specialists, medical students, and residents is constant; they will come and talk to you when you're half awake, just had anesthetic, or when you've just received pain medication. If you don't have someone there to write down this information, write it down yourself, immediately.

- Were treatments and surgery recommended, and by whom? What are the benefits and what are the risks of treatments, testing, and surgery? If you have questions, speak up and ask them and then write the information down. If you think of questions later, write them down and don't hesitate to ask to speak to someone again before the procedure.

2. If a new medication was started, ask what was it and what was the dose? Sometimes a nurse will just show up with a new medication. Don't hesitate to ask:

- Who prescribed it and why? Are there side effects? What are the expected benefits?

- If the nurse doesn't know, or if you need more information, ask to speak to the doctor or to a pharmacist.

   Your "person" can step in when there are concerns and when you are overwhelmed or forgetful:

- "Bob didn't get a chance to tell the anesthetist he has a bad reaction to anesthetics. How do we get that information to them before the surgery?"

- Or, "These don't look like the pills Margaret usually takes. Nurse, would you mind double-checking these are correct?"

The download kit includes checklists for you to print and use, such as a checklist for you to track who came to see you and what they did and recommended, and a medication form.

6. Communication in Preventing Common Medical Errors

Imagine you or your loved one is in hospital. You would do anything to help yourself or them get better. But, in fact, often we remain quiet and become a component of medical error. We are too often concerned about raising a fuss or are embarrassed about saying something to a nurse or a doctor. Our lack of saying something can lead to serious infections, incorrect medications and treatments, and serious progression of a disease.

You and your caregiver can help prevent medical error. If you see something, say something!

Every person involved in your care, including you, has a vital role in preventing medical errors. If you see something that has not been done, if something was done incorrectly, or you are not comfortable with care being provided — you are part of the solution — say something! If the nurse or doctor are not listening or dismissing your concerns, take it higher to a charge nurse, unit manager, or patient complaint office.

6.1 Infection is the number one cause of hospital-induced disease and death

Infection control starts with washing hands — and asking every person who enters your room to wash or sanitize their hands: Gloves are not enough — they need to go over clean hands, changed before caring for every patient, and should be changed during the patient's care if they have been exposed to "dirty" areas during care.

Those with the poorest ongoing record for handwashing are sometimes doctors. If someone is going to touch you, did you see them wash their hands or apply a good dollop of hand sanitizer? If not, speak up. "Hello Dr. Smith, thanks for coming by. I'm probably being a little over-concerned, but did you wash your hands?" I've seen loved ones put a container of hand-sanitizer on the bedside table and merely hand it to every care provider, without saying a word.

6.2 Medication and treatment errors

Nurses and all other staff are to check the patient's bracelet and verify verbally the name and date of birth, every time a medication or other treatment is administered. If you don't see this happen, say something. If that doesn't help, report it!

Errors in giving patients the correct medications, at the right dose, at the right time, by the right route are highly underreported. Errors also occur in taking the wrong blood from the wrong patient.

Make it easy for hospital staff — when someone comes to give you medications, take blood, administer a test, or take you somewhere — hold out your arm with your ID bracelet visible.

Case Study

I was with a patient who had been in the hospital for six months and we were going to an appointment outside the hospital. The transport team came to pick him up and they looked at his ID bracelet and found it completely blank. I asked my client how long it had been since the printing on his bracelet was legible. He told me it had been at least three months. During all that time, it was obvious that not a single nurse had checked his bracelet to make sure he was the right patient to whom they were administering medications. Lab techs had been taking blood and porters had been taking him for tests without verifying he was who he said he was. He said he had told a dozen nurses that his bracelet was no longer legible. I did some quick math, and there was the opportunity for error on at least 300 occasions. I made sure he got a new, legible bracelet immediately, and requested to the unit manager that an incident report be made. (Without incident reports, errors like this are not tracked, reported, or acted upon.)

6.3 Report any change in the status, and stay with the patient if you're looking after someone else

You know yourself and your loved one best. If their pain or behaviour changes — a sudden increase in pain, confusion, or altered level of consciousness — especially sudden and severe confusion, called "delirium" — report it and stay with them until something is done about it.

Note: Sudden and severe onset or spike in confusion is not dementia. While dementia is a slow progression of memory loss and rarely includes hallucinations, delirium is a state often caused by infections or neurological (brain) disorders and should never be dismissed.

Don't be placated (falsely soothed) into believing everything is OK. If the nurse or doctor doesn't take you seriously, go higher on the management chain. This is a really big deal. I've been involved in wrongful death complaints where the family member was concerned and asking for something to be done when they saw a change in their loved one's condition. "If you're told "Don't worry. Why don't you go home and we'll take care of this," this is where you say "No. I appreciate your concern but I will be staying here until I am satisfied that everything with my loved one is OK."

7. Patient Rights in Balance with Patient Responsibility

The most important aspect of being an empowered patient or caregiver is being responsible for your own health and your use of the health-care system (or the health and health-care system use of the person for whom you're caring).

When we are responsible and trying to improve our health, our health-care professionals are likely to respond in kind. If you are perceived as not trying to make things better for yourself, your doctors and nurses are less likely to try and help you. When you are not an active participant in your own care, you may find yourself being ignored or fired because there are so many other patients who are lined up, willing to do the work.

Being responsible for your own body and mind to the greatest degree possible will be rewarded with better health (for example, by losing weight, quitting smoking, exercising more, seeking substance-use treatments — whatever it is that is causing your physical and mental health to suffer). If you care for you, your doctors, nurses, and allied health professionals will often be on board, too.

Sometimes no matter how responsible you are, you still don't receive the care you need. See section 8. for more on this.

Being responsible means trying, wherever possible to be compliant and follow through with recommended treatments and therapies.

On an individual level, we expect everything to be done that can be done for us or a loved one. But on a societal level, we expect patients and the health-care system to be responsible with our tax dollars.

While we all deserve the best health-care possible, and we have all paid for it, there is no pot of health-care dollars with our name on it. Taking care of our own health individually, and being responsible about the health-care services we seek, is the most important thing each of us can do to ensure there are enough health-care dollars for everyone.

8. When You Hit a Communications Wall

If you're already doing all that's being suggested, but you are hitting a wall — or being denied care — strongly consider finding a health-care advocate (a friend or a professional) to help you. Your advocate should meet certain criteria:

- Someone who can attend all physician appointments with you. An educated witness is a very powerful tool. The person you pick should be calm and cool under pressure able to help you sort your thoughts, coach you before and after appointments, and have the self-control to sit back and be as unobtrusive as possible during appointments (if your advocate is overly assertive, he or she may not be invited back).

- Someone who has a basic understanding of the medical system, human anatomy, and physiology.

- Someone who can be a health-care researcher to do some deep digging into your health concerns. Google searches are limited in depth, scope, and credibility. Consider calling a college or university medical library where librarians can help pull up entire medical articles.

- Someone who could help you pick a support group. The group should be supportive and give sound, evidence-based, valid advice.

- A person who can help pick your alternative health-care team (naturopaths, Traditional Chinese Medicine, acupuncturists, etc.) wisely. Too often, the care you receive from them may not be recognized by your Western medicine team. Some functional or integrative clinics have Western doctors on staff and that helps with the transition from one type of health-care paradigm to the other. Use caution when speaking about your alternative treatments to Western medicine doctors: The reaction might be indifference, or skepticism, and you may run the risk of you being labelled difficult. Younger doctors are more likely to be receptive to alternative treatments.

9. Communicating with Dismissive, Arrogant, or Bad Doctors

Despite doing research about our doctors, going in prepared, and having the right level of respectful, assertive attitude, there are occasions when those caring for us are rude, dismissive, or demand our respect rather than earn it. It's tough when you see a doctor who's the opposite of compassionate. When you're sick, you've waited months to see a specialist and you get ten minutes and curt or dismissive responses, it's incredibly frustrating, and it can be devastating.

Great communication skills help. Having an educated witness or advocate with you might make a difference — but sometimes it can make the situation worse. After years of being a navigator-advocate, it is with these difficult doctors that my clients and I have made little headway. There is little to do about this situation except move on by asking for a different specialist. Know that this was not your fault. But do write a report to RateMDs.com, and a letter of complaint to the College of Physicians and Surgeons, so they can monitor and take action so that other patients might be spared the same poor care.

10. Effective Communication Is a Lot of Work, and It's Harder When You're Sick

Having to work so hard when you're sick isn't right and it isn't fair. You want to be treated like you were when you were a sick child: soothed, tucked in, and reassured everything will be all right. It's the one time we don't want to be the adult in the room.

When you're the husband, wife, daughter, son, or friend of the sick or injured person, you likely want to be cared for, too. The additional strain of being proactive and always watching and asking is often just too much. That's when you need someone with you who is assertive and knowledgeable and has your back.

This is your life. You're in charge. Ask for help, as early as you can, rather than hoping things will get better. And, like all things in life, the more we plan, the better the potential outcome.

CHAPTER
THREE
Navigating the Health-Care System

The health-care system and its rules and practices change constantly in an attempt to meet shortfalls and demands. There isn't a week that goes by where a change in policy doesn't directly impact someone. Even when those in the health-care industry have their fingers on the pulse of the system at all levels, it's hard to keep up. How can someone outside of the system be expected to know how it all works?

We call our system fragmented because it is built like puzzle pieces: When put together, it should look like a perfect picture but in reality, it's more like a scrambled box. It is up to you and your team to put that picture together by being empowered patients and caregivers.

We call our system siloed because each portion of the system works distinctly from the others and often, they have little understanding of how the other parts of the system operate. In a large hospital, there are siloes within siloes.

If you have a serious or complex illness, you may need additional help navigating the basics of our complex health-care system.

Develop a support team and consider hiring an independent navigator-advocate before you are in crisis. Refer back to Chapter 1 where I discussed hiring navigator-advocates.

1. How to find a GP or Nurse Practitioner If You Don't Have One

General Practitioners, also known as GPs, Family Physicians, or Primary Care Physicians — or increasingly commonly, Nurse Practitioners (NPs) — are the most important people on your health-care team. They should be the hub, or the quarterback for your care.

There is a critical shortage of GPs and specialists across the country with rural areas and smaller provinces often being hit the worst. There is a push to open more NP-led clinics as a result of this shortage.

Shortages put patients with complex or chronic health problems, and seniors with increasing frailty, in a dangerous place: They are expected to have a GP for testing and referrals, but finding a GP if you're considered complex, elderly, or frail can be a massive challenge as doctors are often reluctant to take on a patient who will take a lot of their already stretched time. Under the College of Physicians and Surgeons' regulations, screening and refusing patients is not allowed but they do it all of the time, often under the guise of a new patient meet-and-greet. There is little enforcement of this regulation.

There is no perfect way to find a new GP or NP except a lot of searching, calling, and door knocking. Here are a few hints:

- See the Resources on the download kit for "Find a Nurse Practitioner" in your province. Often NP led clinics have waiting lists so put your name on it.

- Ask friends and family who their GP is and have them ask if their doctor will take you on as a new patient.

- Some GPs now have wait lists. If you have done you research and want a specific GP, ask if they have a wait list and put your name on it.

- Watch local papers for announcements for new doctors and call immediately.

- Find doctors' offices and clinics in your area and call them regularly to see if they are bringing on new doctors: Sometimes the window to be accepted as a new patient is very short.

- Google "Find a Doctor" + your province. Some provincial College of Physicians and Surgeons, Doctors' Associations, or Primary Care Networks have a list of doctors accepting new patients, but these lists are often out of date and you may still have to do a lot of calling.

- Emergency rooms, urgent care clinics, cancer agencies, and nonprofits such as the Alzheimer's Society, MS Society, etc., may have lists of doctors taking new patients, or may be able to make a referral for you.

Do your homework before seeing a new doctor. Any doctor is not always better than no doctor. In my experience, a bad doctor will overlook vital symptoms, dismiss a patient's concerns (making the patient feel stupid, like a hypochondriac, or small), and may refuse to send the patient for vital referrals and testing. I've reviewed files where bad doctors have directly caused patient deaths. RateMDs.com appears to be the most consistent rating system. Don't stop your search at one negative comment; read on for a consistent picture of compliments and complaints.

1.1 A note about walk-in clinics

If you must use a walk-in clinic, try to be consistent with the clinic you attend. Colleges of Physicians and Surgeons have regulated that patients who attend a clinic regularly, must be assumed to be receiving their primary health care from that clinic and the Canadian Medical Protection Association states, "Provincial/territorial medical regulatory authorities (Colleges) state that patients in walk-in clinics are entitled to care that is the same 'appropriate and professional standard' as in any other setting". (cmpa-acpm.ca, accessed January, 2020).

There is a critical physician shortage across the country. As a patient, do your best to get the care when you need it. Sometimes, your options are not optimal.

2. Improve Care at Appointments

Plan and prioritize what you need to talk about; most doctors' offices announce that they will only address one to two concerns per visit. If you have several things that need to be addressed, it might take some planning.

- If you have several concerns and don't know how to prioritize them, give your doctor a list and ask him or her to help you plan for future appointments.

- Write down what you want to talk about and go over that list before you leave the appointment so you don't miss something important.

- Take your notebook and write notes during the appointment, or immediately following.

- For any appointment where you are getting complicated instructions or information, take someone along with you to take notes and help you ask questions you've forgotten.

- Tell your doctor everything that is relevant. Be truthful, be thorough, and don't skip over something important because it's potentially embarrassing. Your doctor can't make a treatment plan based on incomplete information.

- Use a calendar to plan appointment dates and lab tests — especially when you have multiple upcoming appointments, or they are months away.

3. Get Faster Testing and Referrals to Specialists

Beware the fax machine. One of the advocacy services I offer is to follow up on referrals to specialists and requisitions for testing and we have found that at least one in three referrals or requisitions are not received, don't go to the appropriate specialist, don't have adequate information to be processed in a timely manner, or don't have the correct patient contact information.

You may wait months for a phone call regarding your MRI or CT scan, or your referral to the specialist, and later find out it never arrived.

Unreceived faxes and incomplete information can cost you months of unnecessary wait time and possible progression of your condition. NEVER assume your fax made it to the specialist's office and was handled appropriately.

As an empowered patient or caregiver, be proactive and make sure your referral or requisition went through and is being processed.

For medical testing:

- Wherever possible, ask what was put on the requisition to see if everything you want tested is being tested.

- If your requisition was faxed, find out where your testing requisition was sent to. Give a few days for processing and then call the testing facility and ask if the requisition was received — and, if it's practical for you — that you be put on the cancellation list.

For specialist referrals:

- The more information your doctor puts on the referral form, the better.

  - Specialists triage (prioritize) based on the information they receive.

  - If it's "Urgent" or an "Emergency" for you to see a specialist, ask your GP to make sure that's clear and that there is enough information to support the request. For example, only writing, "abdominal pain" gives the specialist little information. But, "Urgent referral requested: New and sudden of left lower quadrant pain that patient rates as 8/10 on the pain scale. Some bleeding recently noted in stools," will give the specialist much more information and may move you up the list.

- Find out to whom your referral was sent. If you haven't heard anything within a week, check with your doctor to ensure the referral was sent and who it was sent to — even if there is a message that you will be contacted in several months. Or, ask your doctor to confirm it went through.

If your condition worsens, tell your GP and ask that they update your referral. Do not hesitate to call the specialist and let them know about the change in your condition.

4. Improve Care at the Emergency Room

If you've been to an emergency room (ER), you've probably seen the misuse of the system. Due to the shortage of family doctors, patients are resorting (in increasing numbers) to using ERs for urgent, but not emergency care. And, some patients, out of desperation, go to ERs hoping for faster referrals to specialists.

GPs are so often so overbooked that it seems we must plan to be sick, with next-available appointments two to three weeks out.

- If you must see your doctor urgently, let the medical office assistant know why — they often have spaces for urgent same-day appointments.

- Map out your local walk-in clinics and go in early in the day to make sure you can get on the list.

- Is there an Urgent Care clinic in your area? These clinics take serious but non-life-threatening injuries and illnesses. Have their address and phone number on your fridge and phone.

- Emergency rooms are for emergencies! Go there when you have the following:

  - Chest discomfort. For example, pain, heaviness or tightness, shortness of breath, arm pain, neck or jaw discomfort, nausea and heartburn that are unusual or not responding to medication.

  - Neurological changes. For example, signs of a stroke, severe or unusual headache, fainting spells, new onset or change in seizures.

  - Uncontrollable bleeding.

  - Severe and/or sudden pain or rapidly progressing infections (fever, redness, swelling, heat, unusual discharge, red streaks moving upward).

  - All serious injuries and lacerations. All suspected head and neck injuries, and cuts that will require stitches.

If your condition worsens, tell a nurse.

Ways to get faster, more responsive care in an ER:

- Take your medical history, a list of current medications and supplements, and emergency contact information. See Chapter 4.

- Be assertive — not passive and not aggressive. Kindness, respectfulness, and understanding always have a better result than yelling or rudeness.

- Be as clear as possible about your symptoms and concerns. When did your symptoms start? What are they?

- If your condition worsens while waiting for care — or while in care — tell a nurse! **Be assertive!**

- Wherever possible, have someone with you.

- Take a notebook and take notes:

  - Who came to see you?

  - What tests were ordered?

  - What medications were ordered?

  - Is there follow-up you should do?

- Always ask about benefit versus risk for all treatments based on evidence-based medical studies to decide what is best for you.

- Be assertive if you are being discharged and you are concerned your condition is not stable or your concerns were not adequately addressed.

- Be assertive about letting your health team know about any Advance Care Planning wishes and documents.

5. Improve Care in Hospital

- Wherever possible, have someone with you — this is especially important for seniors.

- Take a notebook and document dates and times:

  - The names of all doctors who visit you: specialists, hospitalists (the hospital GPs), and residents.

  - Make notes about recommended changes in care, medications, treatments, and surgeries and their benefits and risks.

5.1 Discharge planning

Unforeseen, early, and inappropriate discharges are the number one reason we are called in as navigator-advocates. Patients have been suddenly told that they will be going home and families are shocked and unprepared. Often, they are not given lists of resources, and home-care assistance will not be available for days to weeks. This can result in patients getting home and then having to go right back to the hospital again.

The only way to prevent this is to be proactive. Be aware that you are likely to be discharged before you're ready. The hospital will be planning for your discharge the moment you're admitted, and you need to do the same. Once you are deemed stable, doctors have little influence on when a discharge will take place. Find out who will make the decision (bed control, a unit manager, etc.) about planned discharge dates and keep following up.

If you are concerned about the success of going home, and you're not getting the information you need, ask for a "Discharge Planning Meeting." The unit Social Worker or Occupational Therapist are often the best people to put together the meeting (but every hospital is a little different). Ask for the following health-care professionals to attend:

- Occupational therapist

- Physiotherapist

- The community care liaison or a community case manager (there are different role titles in every hospital) to discuss home care, rehabilitation, respite, and residential care options

- The Most Responsible Physician (MRP) — often the lead specialist or hospitalist — for your care — for complex discharges with ongoing medical care needs

5.1a What equipment will you need?

- Are there access needs that need to be addressed such as a steep driveway, stairs, narrow hallways, and bathrooms that are not on the same floor as the sleeping area?

- Will a wheelchair fit down hallways and through doorways? (An often overlooked and serious problem.)

- Ask about any special equipment you will need (crutches, cane, walker, wheelchair, shower bench, commode, hospital bed) and where you can rent or buy them.

- If the need for the equipment is temporary and you can't afford it, ask your Occupational Therapist to sign a requisition to get a free equipment loan from your local Red Cross (usually available for a maximum of three months).

- Ask how can you get equipment installed or renovations done.

5.1b Questions to ask about home-care services

- How long will it be until you will be assessed for services when you get home? What will you do until these services are put in place? Do you need to consider private home-care services in the meantime?

- When will home care start? What care needs to be provided in the meantime? Does any training of family caregivers need to be done before discharge?

- What if home is simply not the appropriate choice? Is a rehabilitation unit an option for extra time to recover and get stronger? What does long-term care look like and how long will that process take?

If home is not a safe or viable option, do you need to go into respite (short-term) or residential (assisted living or long-term) care? In most areas, there are long wait lists for these types of housing. You may need to prove the need and why you can't go home with home-care support.

In most provinces there is a "Home First" policy that is in place because, with adequate support, home truly is best, and because there are not enough residential care beds available. But, if you know that you or your loved one cannot manage at home, be assertive and be persistent. Sometimes you will be expected to try being at home and then, if that doesn't work, you'll be put on the residential care list.

In order to get a residential care bed sooner, in a facility of your choice, closer to home, you may want to look at the option of a private pay bed. Ask the social worker or community case manager for lists and options.

6. Transitions of Care – Sometimes Referred to as the Chain of Care

The most vulnerable times for patients are during transitions of care between services. These are the moments when one health-care team has finished their job and the next team has not formally taken over. During the communication handover (often by fax) communication is not always optimal. As empowered patients and caregivers, it is especially important to follow-up with the new care team to make sure all information is received and appointments are confirmed.

Vulnerable transition points:

- Family doctors and Nurse Practitioners to physician specialists: Each looks after their own area of expertise. Communication is often restricted to referral forms and consultation reports that are easily forgotten or lost. Follow up on referrals.

- Emergency rooms to hospital ward: Even when they are in the same building they tend to act like separate planets in a large solar system, each with their own management and specialists. Often nursing reports are phoned from the ER nurse to the nursing unit nurse, and the patient is transported by a porter (a non-medical person). Wherever possible, have someone with you to go over important details with the receiving nurse such as allergies, contact information, advance care planning documents, special personal instructions, to take notes, and follow-up on tests that the ER staff said were to be completed.

- Cancer agencies: A vulnerable point is when ongoing treatments end and palliative and hospice services begin. Confirm that referrals to community care were sent and received.

- Hospital to home and community services: Home health services include home-care, palliative, and hospice services. There are multiple departments within every community health department. Be sure to get contact information and follow-up with community services to ensure that referrals were received, and a case manager will be seeing you as soon as possible.

- Public residential care: Assisted living and long-term care. The weak point is in the first few days to weeks as paperwork is being gathered and care planning begins, and before the team understands the needs and preferences for care for the adult.

Make sure that the ward nurse has had a thorough report and any advance care planning documents.

- Private residential care: These are privately owned and operated but under the rules of the province or health region where they are located. The weak point is during the first few days to weeks as paperwork is being gathered, care planning begins, and before the team understands the needs and preferences for care for the adult. Make sure that they have received the history, consultations, and any advance care planning documents are received and reviewed.

7. Importance of Obtaining and Maintaining your Health-Care Documents

As life goes on, most of us have had medical procedures, operations, and admissions to hospital. If we develop complex and chronic health conditions, the tests and specialist appointments become more frequent. Knowing our own health history is of paramount importance for many reasons, which are discussed in the following sections.

7.1 We forget details and dates

Details and dates that are important to our health-care providers may have slipped from our minds. How many times have you sat in a waiting room with a blank history form, trying to remember surgeries and medical issues and dates? Every time we are forced to use our memories for details, we are likely to forget something important.

7.2 Important documents are often lost or archived

You need to be the keeper of your medical records. Something that happened 20 years ago might be important to your health-care treatments now — but those details are likely long gone from health-care records of doctors' offices and hospitals. And, if your doctor/specialist retires, your records may be stored by a third-party and extremely expensive to retrieve.

7.3 We don't know what's important

For example, our medications may interact with our supplements; what we eat might adversely affect our medications in being effective; a minor reaction to a previous anesthetic, or a parent's severe reaction to an anesthetic, could be relevant for your upcoming surgery. It's important to do a thorough inventory of medications, supplements, past surgeries and medical issues, and then review these with a health-care professional for relevance and level of importance. The free, fillable "In Case of Emergency" form is a good place to start: see Chapter 4. Fill in the form, print it and take it to all of your healthcare appointments.

7.4 We don't know what other doctors and health-team members have reported

If we don't ask for our health records, we can't know or understand what was said in consultation letters: What was said may be incorrect, or it might contain vital follow-up information.

7.5 You are entitled to your health records

Ask the medical office assistant where you attended the appointment for a copy of your consultation. Often your GP can also provide you with a copy. Review the consultation with your GP and ask questions. If follow-up was advised, take note and make sure the recommendations are followed through. If there are errors in the report, you are to request that the author make the changes. (See the College guidelines for the profession and your province.)

7.6 Most of us don't know how to read medical imaging and laboratory reports

Most of us don't know how to read medical reports (and even if we do, we shouldn't be interpreting our own results). It's important to obtain these records but to also review them with your doctor. What may look like an abnormal or worrisome finding to you, may not be as concerning to your doctor, and you need to know why. And, sometimes doctors miss important results and recommendations, and by reviewing these with them, it may flag the need for more investigation.

7.7 Immediate lab results

In some provinces, patients can sign up for immediate access to their laboratory results. In BC and Ontario, see www.myehealth.ca for details. In Alberta, visit https://myhealth.alberta.ca/myhealthrecords. In Saskatchewan, www.ehealthsask.ca.

7.8 Put your documents together

Get a binder, label it, and put it somewhere where it can be easily found (such as on top of or beside the fridge) with your In Case of Emergency documents. See Chapter 4 for details.

- Use binder dividers and sort by: consultations; medical imaging reports; laboratory reports, etc.; and then sort each section by date.

- Do an inventory of what might be missing, make some calls to get copies, and add them to your binder.

- Keep this up as time, testing, and treatments take place.

7.9 Obtain your hospital records

You should obtain your hospital records. You might need them if you —

- were treated in a hospital away from your community hospital and you want your local facility or doctors to have these records for ongoing care,

- are concerned about the care or treatment that you received, or

- want to make a formal complaint or seek legal advice.

Do an electronic search for "Health Records" + the hospital in which you were treated. Download the form, fill in what kind of records you need (for example, consultations and physician progress notes, operating room records, medical imaging and/or laboratory results) and send as recommended in the instructions. Expect that it will take at least 30 business days for your request to be completed.

8. If You Need to Make a Complaint

If there's one part of this book that I hope you don't need to read and act on, it's this one.

We would love to believe that every health-care provider is doing their best work, with the best in mind for their patients, all the time. Unfortunately, it's just not reality. There are a few people in health care (from care aides to doctors) who are burnt out, overworked, or just not suited to the work they have taken on. There are some who are bullies, and a very rare few who derive pleasure from inflicting pain and suffering on the most vulnerable.

There is a very specific order in which to make a complaint regarding care within a hospital or residential care facility. Here are some basic guidelines:

- Try to approach the complaint process as logically as possible. Try to take the emotion out of it: Anger and verbal abuse will inhibit or shut down the process.

- Take the time to take notes with the classic W5 reporting technique:

  - Who was the patient and who was the health-care provider?

  - What happened? Try and give as many details as possible. What did you or your loved one do? Was it reported immediately? What was the outcome when it was reported?

  - Where: Name of the hospital, unit, room, location in room (e.g., bathroom).

  - When: As close to an exact time as possible.

  - Why: Why did it happen? (Examples: state of mind of the patient; state of mind of the health-care provider; was the unit busy; was it understaffed?)

Take notes of anything and everything that was said and done that will jog your mind later. These are your notes and should not be shared with hospital staff: in other words, don't let anyone take your notes and don't allow them to be photocopied.

Unfortunately, as an RN and as a patient advocate, I've witnessed cases of horrendous abuse and neglect. But, it's the smaller, more insidious issues that go under the radar such as preventable infections, medication errors that can cause harm, and even death. As a patient or loved one, it is up to you to stand up for safe and compassionate health care. The more often people report errors, or poor or abusive care, the more professional colleges, hospitals, and governments will be forced to act.

8.1 A special note about assault

If there has been a physical assault on you, your loved one, or another patient, you have the right to immediate action and have the health-care provider removed from the situation. Go through the steps below. If the caregiver is not removed by other staff or managers, you have the right to call the police. Assault is a criminal offence, no matter where it occurs or who the perpetrator is.

8.2 A note of caution about going to the media

Think carefully and logically before contacting the media with your concerns or complaint. It might make you feel better in the short-term, but the repercussions can be significant, especially if your facts are murky, not concise, or worse, inaccurate. Health authorities have staff dedicated to countering media complaints and, though it shouldn't, your public complaint may seriously affect future care of you or your loved one.

8.3 Take a witness

During all meetings, make every effort to have a witness. Your witness should be allowed to take notes, although they may not be able to speak. It's unfortunate, but everyone behaves better, and more honestly, when a third party is in the room. A professional patient or legal advocate is the best person for this role but any calm, logical person is appropriate.

8.4 Complaints about nursing staff (RNs, LPNs, care aides)

Complaints about nursing staff and care aides can include, but are not limited to the following:

- Physical or emotional harm/abuse at the hands of a hospital or residential facility nurse or care aid to you, your loved one, or an assault on another patient you have witnessed.

- Your concerns and complaints regarding symptoms and care were not taken seriously, or not addressed, especially in life-threatening circumstances.

- Care was denied or withheld, especially as a punishment for "bad behaviour" or for speaking up to the care providers.

- When a serious error has taken place and it was not followed up or handled to your satisfaction within the hospital or facility.

- The wrong medications were administered.

- Misidentification of the patient during any treatment, procedure, or surgery.

- Potential transfer of serious pathogen. For example, lack of hand washing or housekeeping exposing you or your vulnerable loved one to bacteria or viruses, especially pathogens that are antibiotic or anti-fungal resistant.

8.5 The complaint process

As calmly as possible, ask to speak to the Charge Nurse: There's one on every shift. Ask to sit in a quiet room. Do not speak openly in a public area, such as the nursing station. If your complaint is not taken seriously and/or is not resolved move on.

- On a day shift, Monday through Friday, ask to speak to the Nursing Manager. They rely on their charge nurses to resolve issues, but you have every right to ask to speak with them if your concern or complaint has not been resolved.

- If the incident occurs on a weekend or on evening (3:00 p.m. to 11:00 p.m.) or during the night (11:00 p.m. to 7:00 a.m.) and only if the situation can't wait until morning, ask to speak with the Nursing Supervisor or Nursing Site Manager. Use your notes and be specific. Why does this require action and resolution right away?

- Ask that an Incident Report be written. This will trigger a review by hospital management.

- If the issue is not resolved fully and to your complete satisfaction, contact the complaints office: The process and department is different for every province and region so do an electronic search for patient complaints + the hospital + your province.

- If you have the name of the nurse or caregiver, you can also make a complaint to the appropriate Nurses' College for your province.

- If the hospital, nursing staff, and complaints office are not responding, or not responding appropriately, and you require immediate resolution, contact your MLA, but be prepared to demonstrate what you've done to resolve this situation on your own.

8.6 Complaints about doctors

Physician care in hospitals: Doctors are not generally employed by the hospital, and their actions (or inactions) within a hospital are not generally mandated or controlled by the hospital. Exceptions are: emergency room physicians, hospitalists, and critical care/intensive care specialists in the larger hospitals. However, all serious incidents and deaths that occur within the hospital are to be reviewed by a special review panel. Doctors are also required to communicate effectively and fully with all other care providers to ensure the best possible outcomes. Any complaints about a physician should go through the hospital complaints process (which should be posted in every hospital) and to the College of Physicians and Surgeons of your province.

Physician care in the community: All concerns and complaints should go to your province's College of Physicians and Surgeons. A link to guidelines for making a complaint are always posted on their websites.

- If the concern is ongoing and affecting your current care, mark the letter as "Urgent and Ongoing Concern."

- Gather as much information as possible (such as consultations and hospital records).

- Have someone with good writing and editing skills review your letter before you submit your complaint.

If you are overwhelmed or angry, if your written communication skills are not the best, or if you have little or no understanding of the health-care system, contact an independent patient advocate for assistance in making your complaint.

CHAPTER
FOUR
In Case of Emergency (ICE): A Form That Communicates When You Can't

Are you prepared for a situation requiring emergency health services or a hospital admission? Help paramedics or hospital staff get important information including:

- Your identity

- Health status

- Medications and supplements

- Life-threatening allergies

- Preference for health-care — especially if you do not want to be resuscitated

- Contact information for people who can speak for you when you can't speak for yourself

It's critical to have accurate, up-to-date information and documentation that can be easily located when minutes matter.

All cell phones have a type of emergency information function that can be accessed without a password (see your phone manufacturer's website for details). Put your basic health and contact information in there. However, this function is minimal, and not all first responders, paramedics, and emergency room staff will look for it.

1. ICE Form

An In Case of Emergency (ICE) Form speaks for you when you are overwhelmed or unable to speak for yourself or a loved one. It has key information about you, your health, and your household, and makes it immediately available to first responders, paramedics, family, and friends.

Patient Pathways has developed an In Case of Emergency (ICE) form that is free, downloadable, and one of the most thorough available. It takes into consideration any advance care planning documents that outline your preferences for future health care and guides your health-care teams to give you the care you want, when you need it. Take a copy of this document to all your doctor and specialist appointments so that your whole health team is on the same page. We are reprinting it here in Sample 1 with permission, and you can access the link to it from the download kit.

In an emergency, time is critical. First responders and paramedics are trained to look for medications and other important health information that could make a life or death difference.

Your fridge is one of the first places first responders are trained to look for this critical information. Basic medical and contact information should be ready and easy to find in an emergency. Post your ICE form and all completed, related documents in a clear plastic zippered folder on the front of your fridge, or in a binder on top of or beside your fridge. If you don't want this information on your fridge, put a clear note on your fridge of where your ICE information can be easily and quickly found.

Note: This information should travel with you to hospital. Give copies of all documents to your appointed health-care representatives and future substitute decision makers.

Sample 1
ICE Form Sample

MEDICAL INFORMATION/IN CASE OF EMERGENCY CALL 911

Full name [Last name, Given names

Personal Health Number

Address

Main phone   Alternate phone

Birthdate [yyyy-mm-dd]

Languages spoken

Date completed [yyyy-mm-dd]

DOCUMENTS INCLUDED WITH THIS FORM:

☐ Legal form naming Substitute Decision Makers *(see instructions)*

☐ No CPR *or* Do Not Resuscitate signed medical order *or* request on Directive *(some provinces require signed medical order)*

☐ Advance/Health Care/Personal Directive or Personal POA *(depending on province)*

☐ Expected Death Form for those nearing end of life, signed by practitioner

☐ Registered Organ Donor **OR** Opted-out of Organ Donation *(for applicable provinces)*

☐ Funeral arrangements and after-death care of body instructions

☐ Enduring Power of Attorney

Other important details can be found:

IMPORTANT CIRCUMSTANCES:

Examples: "I care for my husband Jack. He has dementia and can't be left alone; call his brother Fred," or "Sally has autism and nonverbal," or "I am deaf without my hearing aids."

ICE Form by Patient Pathways. Reproduced by Self-Counsel Press with permission. 2020

In Case of Emergency (ICE) Form

Name	PHN

LIFE THREATENING ALLERGIES:

[Most important and recent at top. Example for *"What to do: Benadryl or EpiPen"*.]

Allergen	
Reaction	What to do

Allergen	
Reaction	What to do

Allergen	
Reaction	What to do

Allergen	
Reaction	What to do

Allergen	
Reaction	What to do

Allergen	
Reaction	What to do

MOBILITY AND SENSORY ISSUES:

- ☐ Paralysis
- ☐ Wheelchair
- ☐ Walker
- ☐ Cane
- ☐ Scooter
- ☐ Others:

- ☐ Prosthetic limb
- ☐ Denture
- ☐ Swallowing
- ☐ Autism spectrum
- ☐ Nonverbal

- ☐ Low/no hearing
- ☐ Hearing aid
- ☐ Low/no vision
- ☐ Eyeglasses
- ☐ Contact lenses

ICE Form by Patient Pathways. Reproduced by Self-Counsel Press with permission. 2020

In Case of Emergency (ICE) Form

Name   PHN

MEDICAL CONDITIONS & RECENT SURGERIES:
[Most important and recent at top.]

Condition

Year diagnosed/
treated   Notes

Condition

Year diagnosed/
treated   Notes

Condition

Year diagnosed/
treated   Notes

Condition

Year diagnosed/
treated   Notes

Condition

Year diagnosed/
treated   Notes

Condition

Year diagnosed/
treated   Notes

Condition

Year diagnosed/
treated   Notes

ICE Form by Patient Pathways. Reproduced by Self-Counsel Press with permission. 2020

Sample 1 – Continued

In Case of Emergency (ICE) Form   Name   PHN

PRESCRIPTION MEDICATION RECORD:
Where these prescribed medications are kept:

☐ Kitchen fridge   ☐ Purse/bag
☐ Bathroom   Other:
☐ Bedroom

Drug				Dosage		
☐ Oral ☐ Ointment	☐ Inhaler ☐ Injection	☐ Patch	When	☐ Morning ☐ Supper	☐ Lunch ☐ Bedtime	
Taken for				Prescribed by	☐ GP ☐ Specialist	

Drug				Dosage		
☐ Oral ☐ Ointment	☐ Inhaler ☐ Injection	☐ Patch	When	☐ Morning ☐ Supper	☐ Lunch ☐ Bedtime	
Taken for				Prescribed by	☐ GP ☐ Specialist	

Drug				Dosage		
☐ Oral ☐ Ointment	☐ Inhaler ☐ Injection	☐ Patch	When	☐ Morning ☐ Supper	☐ Lunch ☐ Bedtime	
Taken for				Prescribed by	☐ GP ☐ Specialist	

Drug				Dosage		
☐ Oral ☐ Ointment	☐ Inhaler ☐ Injection	☐ Patch	When	☐ Morning ☐ Supper	☐ Lunch ☐ Bedtime	
Taken for				Prescribed by	☐ GP ☐ Specialist	

Drug				Dosage		
☐ Oral ☐ Ointment	☐ Inhaler ☐ Injection	☐ Patch	When	☐ Morning ☐ Supper	☐ Lunch ☐ Bedtime	
Taken for				Prescribed by	☐ GP ☐ Specialist	

ICE Form by Patient Pathways. Reproduced by Self-Counsel Press with permission. 2020

In Case of Emergency (ICE) Form

Name   PHN

PRESCRIPTION MEDICATION RECORD — CONTINUED:
Where these prescribed medications are kept:

☐ Kitchen fridge   ☐ Purse/bag
☐ Bathroom   Other:
☐ Bedroom

Drug					Dosage	
☐ Oral ☐ Ointment	☐ Inhaler ☐ Injection	☐ Patch		When	☐ Morning ☐ Supper	☐ Lunch ☐ Bedtime
Taken for					Prescribed by	☐ GP ☐ Specialist

Drug					Dosage	
☐ Oral ☐ Ointment	☐ Inhaler ☐ Injection	☐ Patch		When	☐ Morning ☐ Supper	☐ Lunch ☐ Bedtime
Taken for					Prescribed by	☐ GP ☐ Specialist

Drug					Dosage	
☐ Oral ☐ Ointment	☐ Inhaler ☐ Injection	☐ Patch		When	☐ Morning ☐ Supper	☐ Lunch ☐ Bedtime
Taken for					Prescribed by	☐ GP ☐ Specialist

Drug					Dosage	
☐ Oral ☐ Ointment	☐ Inhaler ☐ Injection	☐ Patch		When	☐ Morning ☐ Supper	☐ Lunch ☐ Bedtime
Taken for					Prescribed by	☐ GP ☐ Specialist

Drug					Dosage	
☐ Oral ☐ Ointment	☐ Inhaler ☐ Injection	☐ Patch		When	☐ Morning ☐ Supper	☐ Lunch ☐ Bedtime
Taken for					Prescribed by	☐ GP ☐ Specialist

Sample 1 – Continued

In Case of Emergency (ICE) Form

Name		PHN

NON-PRESCRIPTION MEDICATIONS, OINTMENTS, & SUPPLEMENTS:

Where these non-prescribed medications are kept:

☐ Kitchen fridge   ☐ Purse/bag

☐ Bathroom   Other:

☐ Bedroom

Drug | **Dosage**

☐ Oral   ☐ Inhaler   ☐ Patch   **When**   ☐ Morning   ☐ Lunch
☐ Ointment   ☐ Injection   ☐ Supper   ☐ Bedtime

Taken for | Recommended by

Drug | **Dosage**

☐ Oral   ☐ Inhaler   ☐ Patch   **When**   ☐ Morning   ☐ Lunch
☐ Ointment   ☐ Injection   ☐ Supper   ☐ Bedtime

Taken for | Recommended by

Drug | **Dosage**

☐ Oral   ☐ Inhaler   ☐ Patch   **When**   ☐ Morning   ☐ Lunch
☐ Ointment   ☐ Injection   ☐ Supper   ☐ Bedtime

Taken for | Recommended by

Drug | **Dosage**

☐ Oral   ☐ Inhaler   ☐ Patch   **When**   ☐ Morning   ☐ Lunch
☐ Ointment   ☐ Injection   ☐ Supper   ☐ Bedtime

Taken for | Recommended by

Drug | **Dosage**

☐ Oral   ☐ Inhaler   ☐ Patch   **When**   ☐ Morning   ☐ Lunch
☐ Ointment   ☐ Injection   ☐ Supper   ☐ Bedtime

Taken for | Recommended by

ICE Form by Patient Pathways. Reproduced by Self-Counsel Press with permission. 2020

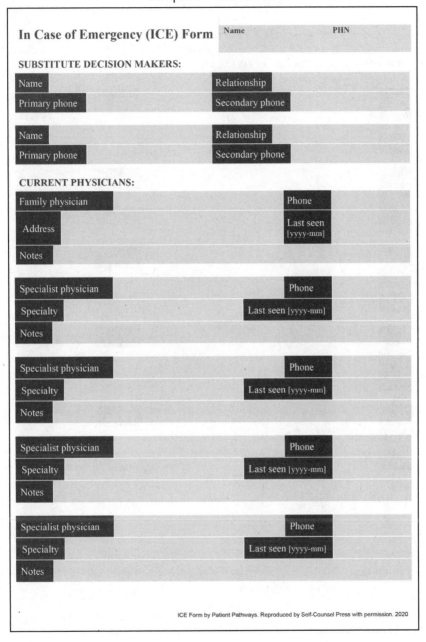

In Case of Emergency (ICE) Form

Name   PHN

SUBSTITUTE DECISION MAKERS:

Name   Relationship

Primary phone   Secondary phone

Name   Relationship

Primary phone   Secondary phone

CURRENT PHYSICIANS:

Family physician   Phone

Address   Last seen [yyyy-mm]

Notes

Specialist physician   Phone

Specialty   Last seen [yyyy-mm]

Notes

Specialist physician   Phone

Specialty   Last seen [yyyy-mm]

Notes

Specialist physician   Phone

Specialty   Last seen [yyyy-mm]

Notes

Specialist physician   Phone

Specialty   Last seen [yyyy-mm]

Notes

ICE Form by Patient Pathways. Reproduced by Self-Counsel Press with permission. 2020

In Case of Emergency (ICE) Form

Name   PHN

PERSONAL AND HOUSEHOLD CONTACTS:
[Examples: *"Building manager, friend with key"*]

Name		Phone
Role		
Notes		

Name		Phone
Role		
Notes		

Name		Phone
Role		
Notes		

Name		Phone
Role		
Notes		

Name		Phone
Role		
Notes		

NOTES

ICE Form by Patient Pathways. Reproduced by Self-Counsel Press with permission. 2020

Review all of your documents at least once a year or when any of the following happen:

- Any medication changes
- A change in diagnosis or health status
- A hospitalization
- A change in your Substitute Decision Maker
- A serious diagnosis or death of a loved one

If you are not using our form, we recommend that you gather the following information for your ICE document:

- Date completed
- Full name
- Date of birth
- Health-care number
- Address
- Phone number(s)
- Primary language spoken
- Documents included (if applicable):
  - Substitute Decision Maker documents
  - "No CPR or DNR" orders
  - Advance directive
  - Expected Death in the Home
- Where other important documents can be found
- Important circumstances. This identifies critical and immediate information for first responders and hospital staff. Some examples might be: "I care for my husband Jack. He has dementia and can't be left alone; call his brother Fred," or "Sally has autism and is nonverbal," or "I am deaf without my hearing aids."

- Life-threatening allergies, reactions, and treatments (and after those, non-life-threatening allergies and sensitivities).

- Mobility and sensory issues: For example: you might be legally blind but still need your glasses; or you need a cane or a walker to walk.

- Medical conditions and recent surgeries.

- Current and recent illnesses, conditions, and treatment information:

  - Medical conditions should be listed from the most serious to the least serious, for example: diabetes, dementia (what stage), congestive heart failure, high blood pressure, cancer (what type and where), etc.

  - List surgeries from your most recent: for example: gallbladder removal, Jan 2019; open heart surgery, 2015; tonsillectomy, age 5.

  - List any implants that you have, for example: pacemaker, automatic defibrillator, hip replacement, etc.

- Prescription medications: List all medications you take and frequency, and where you keep your prescription medications. You can also ask your pharmacist to print a list of your current prescribed medications each time you get new ones.

- Non-prescription medications, ointments, and supplements: Many supplements and over-the-counter medications can react with prescribed medications. Be sure to list them all.

- Substitute decision makers: These are the people you want to speak for you when you can't speak for yourself in an emergency. They are the people that you have chosen as your substitute decision makers, and who have had conversations with you about what you would want if a health crisis or catastrophe happens. They are not the people who help you out with pet care, picking up the mail, or watering the lawn. List these people under Personal and Household Contacts.

- Current physicians and health-care providers: List your family doctor and any specialists that you are currently or have recently seen.

- Personal and household contacts: These are the people you might need to have someone call (for example, the hospital social worker) if you are in hospital for an unexpected or extended stay. This may include caregivers for other family members, pet care providers, someone to pick up the mail or empty the fridge, garden help, etc.

2. Review and Update Your Information Regularly

Review this information and make updates whenever your health or personal circumstances change. Put a copy on your fridge; keep a copy in your wallet and/or have a copy in your phone documents; and give a copy to all your physicians, as this form will be more thorough than most of their history forms.

CHAPTER
FIVE
Financial Planning for Serious Illness, Injury, and Disability

None of us, no matter our age, wants to think about the financial impact of serious illness and injury. But not thinking about it and not planning for it can have devastating results. You don't have to have a large income and savings to make proactive, important decisions.

Contrary to widely held beliefs, health care is not free in Canada and it is getting more expensive every day. Our doctors' appointments, most testing, hospitalizations, and some treatments are covered under our health-care plans, but little else is. Many health expenses are covered or subsidized by employers or private extended benefits insurance — but these benefits frequently end when we retire and are entering our most expensive health-care years. Those with low incomes may have a portion of their medications covered under a provincial program.

If you have a financial planner, talk to him or her not only about retirement planning but also illness and injury financial protection. This chapter is not meant to substitute the advice of an experienced financial planner, but to give you a realistic glimpse of the financial challenges Canadians face when they become seriously ill or injured.

There are different financial challenge for every age group especially for those who are self-employed or stay-at-home parents. The following are some things to think about no matter your age or stage of life.

1. Common Health Expenses Not Covered by Provincial Health Plans

There are many medical expenses not covered by individual provinces' health plans. This can cause further anxiety for those impacted by serious illness or injury. If possible, plan and save for the future. If you are nearing retirement, find out if you can take over and pay for your own extended benefits. Some insurers allow you to sign up for an extended benefits retirement policy within 60 days of your last day of work, so do your research and learn about the options available to you.

Some lower costs (that can really add up):

- Accommodation for patients and family away from home for treatment
- Ambulance and hospital transfers
- Taxi rides to and from treatments
- Meals at hospitals
- Parking at hospitals and medical offices

Medium-sized costs:

- Time off or reduced income for family and caregivers
- Private and semi-private hospital rooms if requested and NOT needed for nursing reasons (i.e., infection isolation)
- Medications not covered by Pharmacare that can't be ordered by a specialist under Special Authorization (generally newer drugs)
- Medical equipment such as walkers and home safety items
- Publicly subsidized residential care fees based on yearly income (not assets)

High costs:

- Medical equipment such as wheelchairs and home renovations
- Private Pay Residential Care
- Assisted Living Residential Care
- Independent Living
- Private in-home nursing care
- International surgery; $25,000 to $100,000 or more

2. Financial Planning for Those Who Are Still Working: Adults 18 to 65

Most adults 18 through 65 who are still working rarely think about illness or injury and the resulting impact on income and assets. The majority of us have not done basic homework on our employment benefits. It's scary to think about being unable to work due to serious illness or injury so we simply choose not to look at the repercussions of the sudden loss or decrease in income.

Sick people often end up being poor people.

Financial stress can cripple and destroy families.

Imagine that you are still employed and are suddenly critically ill or injured. The care you receive in hospital is free but your income suddenly stops. You might have sick time, or short-term or long-term disability coverage from work, but there are a lot of forms and paperwork to fill out — which is hard from a hospital bed — and there might be a significant wait for your first cheque. You might be shocked that disability payments are most often taxable and generally 66 percent of your previous income. You might also want or need your spouse to take time off work to help care for you. Or, maybe an adult child will need to take time away from work to be by your side. The bills and the stress begin to mount.

Carrie is a 35-year-old Registered Nurse. Two years ago, she developed a severe autoimmune disease and had to quit work. At the beginning of her illness she had very few sick days available (she admitted that she had sometimes used these for minor illnesses or mental health days) and she had no savings because she was still paying off student loans. She applied for Employment Insurance sick benefits that capped out, after taxes, at less than 50 percent of her regular take-home wage. Then there was a two-month gap between her EI finishing and her long-term care disability kicking in. During that period, she was forced to go on Social Assistance and move into her parents' basement suite. And, now, two years later, her disability insurer is saying there is not enough evidence to say she is substantially disabled and they are forcing her to find a position in any job and will be cutting her off benefits.

2.1 Benefits packages

It is vital to understand your benefits package, especially disability and extended benefits clauses. It means looking deeper than the glossy package handed out by Human Resources (HR). If you are in an association or union, look at your contracts for wording and entitlements. Or ask your HR department for your entitlements and if they don't know, ask them to contact the insurer for detailed information.

- Disability benefits: What is the percentage of your income you can expect to see? Is this income taxable, and when do benefits begin?

- Extended benefits coverage: When you are sick or injured, you will need these benefits more than ever. But some policies are limited in how long your benefits will be in force. If your extended benefits will end, find out if you can continue to pay the premiums, and what the deadline is to take them over.

If you have sick days and they are bankable, save them, wherever possible. You might need them to cover the period between sick time, short-term disability, and/or long-term disability.

Will you have a financial shortfall if you're on disability leave? Can you manage your month-to-month expenses on 66 percent, or less, of your current wage? If not, start saving money for the top-up and plan for a minimum of six months.

- Talk to a financial planner about buying private disability insurance that will top up financial shortfalls. If you purchase your own disability insurance, the payments you receive will be tax-free.

- Consider buying a comprehensive Critical Illness policy that will pay out a tax-free lump sum, depending on the policy, on 3 to 23 serious illnesses or injury diagnoses upon 30 days after diagnosis. The younger you are when buying this policy, the more affordable it is. You can get a Return of Premium policy where your funds are returned to you at age 65 if you have not made a claim.

2.2 For the self-employed

It is important for self-employed people to talk to their accountants and financial advisors about income and then consider purchasing disability insurance. Those who are self-employed often write off as many expenses as possible to reduce their taxable income — but that can backfire when it comes to disability benefits. Disability insurance is based on your income, reducing the amount you receive while off on disability.

Some tips:

- Look into group extended benefits and disability plans through organizations such as the Chamber of Commerce.

- Consider buying a comprehensive Critical Illness policy. These policies are not based on income. A tax-free lump sum on 3 to 23 (depending on the policy) serious illnesses or injury diagnoses pays out 30 days after diagnosis. The younger you are when buying this policy, the more affordable it is. You can get a Return of Premium policy where your funds are returned to you at age 65 if you have not made a claim.

- Inquire with Workers Compensation and Employment Insurance if you are eligible to make voluntary payments so you are eligible for benefits in case of injury or illness.

2.3 For those who have a low reportable income or if you are a stay-at-home spouse

Katie was a 52-year-old mother of two teenage boys and she was a stay-at-home mom. She was healthy and vibrant and worked without a wage coordinating her husband Max's business. As such, she was an active partner in the family's income generation. But, according to Canada Revenue Agency, she had no income.

Within a month of her 53rd birthday, her health, and their lives, turned upside down. Katie was admitted to hospital for a severe headache. She was having a massive stroke. Her hospitalization and rehabilitation took over a year. She was eventually able to go home but she was paralyzed on her right side, she would always need to be in a wheelchair, and she would always need physical support.

Max had to take time off from his busy business to be at her side and assume all of the duties his wife had done effortlessly: business paperwork, driving the kids to all of their activities and being cheerleader at their games, providing meals (he had never cooked) in the midst of chaotic schedules, shopping, and cleaning their large home.

His business suffered. He needed to hire a cook and a housekeeper, just to keep from drowning. Max was eventually able to regain his emotional and financial footing, but he estimates that he lost at least $100,000 in the year after Katie's health crisis due to lost earnings and replacement of household services.

Financial preplanning options are limited when a person is not generating income but there were two financial planning scenarios that Max and Katie could have put into place prior to her illness:

- A savings account specifically to cover serious illness. Financial planners have calculation tools to help you figure out how much you and your family might need to save to cover wage losses and extra services that might be needed (generally for six months to a year).

- Critical illness insurance is a lump-sum payment for an amount you choose that is paid 30 days after the diagnosis of a serious, life-altering, or threatening injury or illness. The person being covered does not need to be employed or have a large income. It is a great option for stay-at-home parents or those who are self-employed. It can be used to top-up disability plan income shortfalls. The money can be used for anything you see fit.

3. Our Most Expensive Health Years Are after 65

If you're reading this, and you are older than 55 years of age, it's time to do advance care and financial planning.

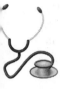

"Isn't it funny that many of us tend to take out life insurance in case we die prematurely but don't make provisions for the very likely possibility that we'll need care? I doubt you look forward to your care home stay, the tightly scheduled visit of the district nurse, or the look on the face of your children when they need to decide whether they want to sell the house they grew up in to pay for better care for you.

"... It's not to say that governments and healthcare providers shouldn't take responsibility for care – they do anyway – but if we blindly rely on them to provide, there are limits to what we will receive. Before it's too late, it's better that we also come up with plans of our own." (Dr. Anna Schneider in "We Took a Snapshot of the Last Year of People's Lives – Here's What We Found," TheConversation.com, accessed October, 2019).

As we age, our paperwork is often the first thing to suffer. Take the time early in your retirement years to get your paperwork in order and do your best to keep it up to date. It is not uncommon for people acting as Enduring Powers of Attorney and Executors to give up almost as soon as they start when they see the mess they need to sort through.

- Get and keep your paperwork and accounts in order and let your decision makers know where these documents can be found.

- Review your financial and legal documents with your Enduring Power of Attorney.

- If possible, save and set aside adequate funds that can easily be turned into cash.

- Do not rely on being able to sell your home to finance illness, injury, or living expenses.

- For a serious illness or injury, if you can afford it, a professional navigator-advocate can help you save money, time, and stress.

Our golden years are likely to be the most expensive years of our lives and most of us don't plan for them adequately. Our income is often fixed and families are often forced to take lines of credit or sell their homes to pay for medical equipment or private care.

Over the last seven years, I have seen a critical and frightening decline in the availability of subsidized health care. Home care is now in crisis; there are not enough qualified caregivers and there is not enough funding; residential care waitlists for adults who qualify, nearly always because of advancing dementia, can be one to two years long. Adults are expected to liquify their assets to assist in paying for private home care and residential care. And, families are often expected to help pay for these services, too.

Being proactive about your paperwork and finances can go a long way in preventing financial crisis as you age.

4. Powers of Attorney (POAs) and Enduring Powers of Attorney (EPOAs)

An Enduring Power of Attorney (EPOA) is different from a Power of Attorney (POA). To create either document, you must be the legal age of majority, and mentally capable. A POA is in effect only when you are mentally capable; it immediately ends when you become mentally incapable. An EPOA is in effect when you are mentally incapable (which includes many situations while in hospital). It can also be in effect when you are mentally capable.

An Enduring POA document may not state the word "enduring" in its heading. Read the body of the document for the words, "while capable or incapable."

You can use EPOA and POA documents to appoint one or more people to be your "attorney" to handle your financial and legal affairs. (Attorney does not mean lawyer in this case. Most people appoint a spouse, family member, or friend in a POA or an EPOA.)

You can restrict your attorney's authority to specific dates or tasks.

You can use an EPOA to appoint one or more people to handle your financial and legal affairs.

For Advance Care Planning, an Enduring Power of Attorney is recommended: Your EPOA may need to provide your CRA Notice of Assessment for home care or residential (long-term) care subsidy benefits.

4.1 When do you need an EPOA?

You need an EPOA if —

- you own property,

- you have investments or money that needs to be managed, or

- money is needed from your accounts to pay for living expenses and regular bills.

Note: You can put together a simple EPOA without a lawyer or notary public but strongly consider the services of a professional lawyer and/or accountant if any illness (expected or not) may require complex transfers of funds or sale of assets to pay for your care, pay bills, or run a business. It is also important to understand the tax consequences of the transfer or sale of your assets.

Plan carefully before making any decisions about your financial affairs. Get quotes and fees from any and all third-party financial planners, lawyers, and/or trust companies.

Think deeply about who the best and most trustworthy person would be to be your EPOA.

Unless a specific trigger as to when the EPOA is activated is stated in the document, a Power of Attorney or an Enduring Power of Attorney is effective immediately. This grants your POA access to all your financial and legal affairs and gives them an extraordinary amount of power over your life. It should be someone you trust and who will put your best interest first. Carefully consider who you choose and include details about when you want the EPOA to be in effect.

Your POA/EPOA can liquidate assets and sell your home without you knowing it. Too often, they can use your investments and bank accounts as their own piggy bank.

See *Power of Attorney*, another Self-Counsel Press title for more information, or consult your lawyer.

5. Elder Financial Abuse

Elder financial abuse is shockingly common. If you have ANY reservations of having one of your adult children, relatives, or friends as your Enduring Power of Attorney, strongly consider having an independent Trust Company assume this responsibility. Their fees often pale in comparison to the headaches — sometimes nightmares — that can result.

PART

TWO

Advance Care Planning: Why and How to Use It

In the second part of this book, we will discuss how to –

- choose future decision makers in case of serious injury, illness, and incapability – a person who will speak for you when you can't speak for yourself;

- explore your values and beliefs;

- determine where you are in your health journey;

- learn tools to have vital, ongoing conversations about advance care planning;

- write a detailed advance directive; and

- consider options for end-of-life possibilities.

CHAPTER
SIX
Advance Care Planning: Definition and Conversations

Advance care planning is an umbrella term for ongoing conversations and documentation about your values, beliefs, and preferences for care when you are seriously injured or ill, or for when you have been diagnosed with a life-threatening or life-ending illness.

The Advance Care Planning Umbrella as seen in Figure 1 gives an overview of all the areas encompassed by this topic.

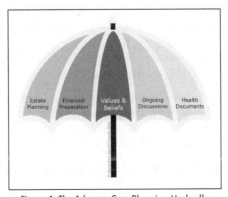

Figure 1: The Advance Care Planning Umbrella

Estate planning includes:

- Life insurance

- Business planning and insurance

- Trusts

- Wills and executors

The **financial preparation** part of it includes considering:

- Health insurance: short- and long-term disability, critical illness, and long-term care

- Getting and keeping financial documents in order

- Enduring Powers of Attorney

- Agreements

- Investments and retirement planning

- Liquid assets to pay for unforeseen costs of loss of income, medical equipment, and private home care and private residential care

We also need to consider **values and beliefs, and preferences for future health care**:

- Think about what's important in our lives now and for serious injury, illness, and end-of-life.

- Determine where you are in your health journey.

Also, there are **ongoing conversations** that will need to be had that include:

- Over the natural course of our lives, having conversations with those we love and those who will care for us about our values, beliefs, and future wishes for health-care.

- Writing letters to loved ones.

- Having frank conversations with our health-care team about our health journey, values, and beliefs.

There is **health documentation** to take care the following:

- Medical history and In Case of Emergency documentation.

- Choose Substitute Decision Makers, informally or formally.

- Write an informal or formal advance directive clearly stating your wishes for health care.

- End-of-life documents: No CPR or DNR orders; MAiD document; Expected Death at Home.

Advance care planning (ACP) starts with conversations and documentation that are directly applicable to your health care. ACP ends the moment you die.

Estate planning includes documentation in preparation for the management and disbursement of your assets after you die. Estate planning ends the moment of your death when estate administration begins.

Both advance care planning and estate planning can only take place while you are still capable or competent.

Advance care planning is for all adults of all ages and all stages of health. The earlier we begin these conversations, and the planning that goes along with it, the more natural, less scary, and less fraught with emotion this process is. It's important to regularly review and make changes as your circumstances change.

Advance care planning is preparation for serious injury and illness at any age.

Life-altering illness and injury can happen at any age. In fact, those who are younger than the age of 50 are most likely to have sudden, catastrophic illnesses and injuries that can lay ruin to finances and families.

When we are still healthy, we assume everything that can be done will be done to save us and bring us back to health. But, what about the time in between illness and health? What have you put in place financially for that period when you might not be able to manage, physically and mentally, and who will help care for you and help make vital decisions? See Chapter 5 about finances.

If you are reading this book because you are a caregiver for someone else, think of this as an opportunity for your own self-work around advance care planning.

This process becomes imperative when you are dealing with —

- one or more chronic illnesses,

- a complication from chronic disease,

- dementia,

- having trouble caring for yourself, or

- a life expectancy of less than one to two years.

1. The Advance Care Planning Process

Each of the following parts of advance care planning is broken down in the following chapters:

1. Decide on who will be your future decision makers, referred to as Substitute Decision Makers (SDMs): Decide on who are the best people to speak for you and make important decisions for you if you are no longer capable (Chapter 7).

2. Determine your values and beliefs (Chapter 8).

3. Determine where you are in your health journey (Chapter 9).

4. Document your wishes for future health care: Advance Directive (Chapter 10).

5. Vital, ongoing conversations: with your loved ones, substitute decision makers, and your health-care team. (Chapter 11).

6. Considerations for End of Life (Chapter 12).

Note that every province has a different name for the formal legal health directive document. We are using the term advance directive because it is becoming the standard term around the world. You will find the name of the document for your province and any specific requirements for writing it, in Chapter 10.

Your values, beliefs, and preferences for future health are likely to change with progression of serious illness and age. Keep in mind these cues to re-examine your ACP documents:

- If you have a new diagnosis or a change in diagnosis.

- When your representative moves, becomes ill, or dies.
- When your health changes.
- When five years have passed since you last updated your documents.
- After the death of someone who is significant in your life.
- If your marital status changes.

2. The Importance of Advance Care Planning and Dementia

A special note about the importance of advance care planning for those with dementia: It really does seem too soon until it's too late.

It is difficult — and important — to have these discussions as soon as possible when any type of dementia is suspected — because they can only take place during the early stages of decline. As the disease progresses, it will be more difficult to express your wishes. As a loved one, you may need to be the one to start this conversation.

We often hesitate because it may seem unkind to suggest to the person we love that they are losing their mental ability. We are often afraid when we see the clues, see the symptoms, and then hear the diagnosis. It's normal to be held back by our own fear of the future, afraid of loss, and what will happen.

We may feel alone. And we may fear that our loved one's response would be denial, anger, or depression. It's tempting to postpone the talk until tomorrow, or the next doctor's appointment, or after the holidays. It seems easier to talk around the person, to pretend that the memory loss is normal at his or her age, and to join in a conspiracy of denial.

2.1 Opportunities for conversation

When your loved one expresses concerns about their memory loss, use this as an opportunity to listen and open discussions. Keep discussions short and simple and be open to further discussions as they come up.

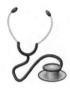

For more on having conversations, go to the Conversation Project –
Your Conversation Starter Kit: Institute for Healthcare Improvement:
https://theconversationproject.org/wp-content/uploads/2017/02/
ConversationProject-StarterKit-Alzheimers-English.pdf.

The following case studies show how all the pieces of the advance care planning umbrella go together.

Case Study

Michelle is 38 years old. She is a married professional with two young children. She found a breast lump two weeks ago and has just had an emergency lumpectomy and lymph node biopsy, showing moderately aggressive stage-three cancer.

With chemotherapy and radiation, there is a good chance she will be cancer-free. But she began thinking about what she wants for herself, and her family, if the cancer comes back.

Estate planning: She had purchased a life-insurance policy several years before – and that's important because with a diagnosis of cancer, she would no longer qualify. She has updated her will and made provisions for the care of her children, should something also happen to her husband.

Financial planning: Michelle has disability insurance through her work and a private critical-illness insurance policy which will be paid to her in another two weeks. She is not worried about her financial future and is able to focus on treatment and recovery. She has joint bank accounts with Rob and all of their assets are in both of their names but she will get an Enduring Power of Attorney assigned to Rob to ensure there are no issues with their finances.

Values and beliefs: Michelle values her family above all else. She is ready and willing to try any and all treatments in order to stay alive, well, and healthy so she could see her family grow up. She values her husband Rob's input and they talk regularly about their hopes, dreams, and fears. They seek counselling to keep lines of communication open.

Assigning Substitute Decision Makers: Rob is automatically her SDM, but she formalized that with a legal document, and also named her sister, Terri, to be a formal SDM to make decisions with Rob, and allow her to make decisions independently of Rob if he was unable to make decisions.

Advance directive: She states she wants to be resuscitated and everything done to keep her alive. She will revisit this if her disease progresses.

Debbie is 65 years old. She is healthy and active. Her mother, Maureen, is 92 years old, in long-term care, and has had a series of small strokes and is being treated for a bout of pneumonia but is not getting better. Debbie was called by the doctor to discuss changing her mother's resuscitation orders from "active medical treatment" to end-of-life "comfort care." Debbie needed more information and attended an advance care planning session. While there, she was encouraged to do her own advance care planning.

Values and beliefs: It was tough for Debbie to see her once-vital mother slowly decline and become dependent on others for everything, including eating. Debbie values her own independence above all else and wants to avoid going down the same road as her mother. She has adult kids and grandchildren of her own who she wants to be around for and will work at staying healthy and fit for as long as possible.

Vital conversations: Debbie close to meet individually with all her loved ones. She tells everyone she's perfectly healthy, and fully intends to live for a long time, but that she's being proactive and that if something sudden and serious happens to her, what she wants the rest of her life to look like – and not look like. She lets her doctor know that she's begun her ACP conversations and they set a plan to review her documents if her health changes.

Assigning Substitute Decision Makers: Both of Debbie's adult children live out of town. They also have very busy lives with their jobs and families. She assigns formal documentation naming her cousin, Bev, as her primary SDM, and her brother, Mac, as alternative. However, she will write in her Advance Directive that, wherever possible, she wants her SDMs to consult with her adult children and that any end-of-life planning should be done as a team.

Advance directive: She states that if she were to have a sudden, serious injury or illness and she could no longer speak for herself, she would want to be resuscitated but she would want her prognosis to be reviewed. If there was a good chance she would require assistance for daily activities – especially if it was likely she would need to be in residential care – that she wanted life-support to be removed and to let infections take its course.

She will review and update her Advance Directive regularly, especially if her health changes.

Financial planning: Debbie has just retired. She qualified for retirement extended benefits and applied for those the moment she retired. She has begun to withdraw her pension and CPP. She has some funds that she can easily liquidate in case of a sudden health crisis. She has assigned her daughter to be her enduring power of attorney.

Estate planning: She has assigned her daughter to be her enduring power of attorney and assigned both of her adult children to be her executors. She has life insurance in place until she is 100.

Jerry was 62 years old when he was diagnosed with ALS. He was single, but had a close relationship with his niece, Teresa who lived nearby, and had a few close friends. He was ready and willing to try everything to slow the neurological progression of the disease. He was angry and wasn't ready to look at the possibility of dying. It took time and conversations with his doctors, his ALS mental health support team, and ALS patient support groups before he was able to look at his mortality.

Six months after his diagnosis with ALS, Jerry's neurological symptoms were worsening. With support, he began his homework and reflection on what was important to him as he neared the end of his life.

Values and beliefs: It became clear to Jerry that his values were time with his friends, good meals, conversation and laughs, and he wanted to stay as independent as possible. He still wanted everything done for him should he have a health crisis. He didn't want to suffer and he didn't want to be dependent on others. He wanted to die rather than go into residential care.

Vital conversations: First, he talked to Teresa about his diagnosis, prognosis, and what he wanted for the rest of his life, and at the end of his life. He talked to her about having Medical Assistance in Dying (MAiD). It was an emotional talk for both. Then he talked to his friends and told them how important it was that they help him live life as normally as possible and continue their outings and activities as long as possible. He talked to his GP and specialists about his prognosis and asked that they be honest and straightforward with him as diagnosis progressed. He got a palliative care team in place.

Assigning Substitute Decision Makers: Teresa agreed to be his SDM and they put formal paperwork in place.

Advance directive: It was tough work for Jerry to look at his life in clinical terms and he put this off as long as possible. A bout of pneumonia and a near-miss with needing to go on a ventilator, pushed the decision. He wrote a detailed plan, knowing it would have to be revised frequently as his disease progressed. For now, he still wanted everything done.

Financial planning: Jerry had a trust company assigned as Enduring Power of Attorney and Executor. He knew this could be a big job and didn't want to put it on his niece or his friends.

Estate planning: The trust company began to work with Jerry on pre-planning and organizing his estate.

Max is 71 years old. He was diagnosed with mild hypertension (high blood pressure) at the age of 58 and has been on a mild diuretic (water pills) since then. At age 63 he was diagnosed with diabetes. He now has mild kidney failure and has developed angina, and both are being treated successfully with medication and lifestyle changes, including a better diet and regular exercise. He feels and looks well and his doctors are just keeping an eye on things.

Despite his doctors' reassurances, Max realizes that health issues are starting to add up. Even though he feels and looks well all of this has been a bit of a wake-up call. When he was honest with himself, he knew that he was no longer a spring chicken. His father died of a heart attack in his mid-70s and his mother had a long road with dementia and he knew he didn't want to linger like she did. He began the process of looking at his values and beliefs.

Values and beliefs: He knew that quality of life with his wife, children, and grandchildren was more important to him than life at all costs. He would do everything he could to restore and maintain his health but he was also going to keep asking questions about the risks versus benefits of future treatments. He did the exercises on determining what was important to him, with his wife, Jill. (She began her own advance care planning.) They started a bucket list and decided to get serious about checking things off.

Vital conversations: Talking to Jill was easy but, his adult children, not so much; one of his sons got up and left the room and said he wouldn't talk about it again. But, he did talk to his other kids, mostly about what he didn't want if his health went sideways. The toughest conversation was with his GP, who thought the conversation was much too premature, but Jerry pushed forward and finally had constructive conversations.

Assigning Substitute Decision Makers: Jill was clear that she didn't feel comfortable about receiving health information or making hard medical decisions – she simply wanted to be his wife if he was seriously ill. He assigned his eldest son, Mark, to be his formal SDM, because he lived the closest.

Advance directive: Jerry decided he didn't want CPR done, unless he was already in hospital. But he did want everything else done, unless it didn't look like he wouldn't bounce back.

Financial planning: He put paperwork in order, consulted with his financial advisor and accountant, and named his daughter as EPOA.

Estate planning: With all his paperwork in order, he reviewed his will, which was still valid.

CHAPTER
SEVEN
Choose Who Will Speak for You When You Cannot Speak for Yourself

No one should be alone in the health-care system! If you experience serious injury, illness, or advancing dementia, you may not be able to speak for yourself. That makes it the most vulnerable time in your life. The health-care system moves fast and with a constant turnover of doctors and nurses, communication is often not what it should be. You will need someone to be at your side and to speak for you.

Max was 71 years old when he did his estate and advance care planning, naming his wife as his legal SDM and his son Mark (who lived the closest) as his alternate. Max is now 78 and was recently diagnosed with four heart blockages that required a quadruple open-heart bypass. But his wife had medical issues of her own and wasn't capable of being at Max's side. Mark stepped in as his legal SDM.

Prior to Max's surgery, he talked to Mark again about his values and beliefs. He wanted everything done for him during the surgery but if things went wrong, Mark would be able to step in and make Max's wishes known.

1. What If You Are Alone?

More than 4 million Canadians live by themselves, a dramatic increase since the 1980s. For those who have adult children, they are often spread out, and they may not have frequent contact with them.

When we live alone, our friendships become even more important. Some of us don't have close friends or neighbours to ask to be at our sides at medical appointments and during hospitalizations.

If you're truly alone, there are things you can do to protect yourself while receiving health care:

1. Be extra vigilant in taking the time to gather your health history and have an In Case of Emergency form prepared and on your fridge.

2. Take thorough notes during all health-care appointments and hospitalizations.

3. Work at developing relationships with others — because there are so many upsides to developing friendships — and with time and growing trust, reach out to friends to be your substitute decision makers.

4. Consider hiring a professional health-care navigator-advocate to be by your side.

2. Choose Who Will Speak for You

The person who speaks for you is called your Substitute Decision Maker (SDM). This person is someone you ask and assign, informally or formally. Most of us assume that someone, anyone, is going to show up, be at our side, and help us make vital health-care decisions. Most often we are assuming that our spouse or our adult children will be there. Sometimes that's an adequate plan but it comes with its risks.

You may not want the person on the legal hierarchy (see section 2.1) speaking for you, if you are not able to speak for yourself. You might be in conflict with them or they may act on their own values and beliefs rather than your own.

Not everyone is good in a health-care crisis and sometimes they're not available — and because of that, you may not have someone at your bedside, overseeing your care, asking important questions and gathering vital information, or voicing your values, beliefs, and preferences for care in a critical situation. How to decide on who would be the best person to make decisions for you is discussed in the next section.

Debbie was 62 years old when she wrote up her SDM documentation. When she was 70 years old, her husband died. Her two adult children were living out of province and both had young families. It would be a financial hardship for her children to fly to her side and take time off work. So, Debbie rewrote her documentation to make her best friend, Beth, her decision maker. She wrote in her advance directive that Beth was to consult with both of her adult children regarding any health-care decisions but Beth was to be the spokesperson.

2.1 Legal hierarchy of Substitute Decision Makers

By not choosing your Substitute Decision Makers (SDMs), if you become incapable of choosing someone — the medical system will choose that person based on a provincially legislated hierarchy.

The person must have been in contact with you within the last 12 months. Most provinces state you must have been on good terms and no conflict with this person. Here is the order from top to bottom:

- Spouse, including common-law (generally after one year of cohabitation)
- Adult child or children (if more than one child, they are to assign a spokesperson and make decisions together)
- Parents or guardians
- Siblings (if more than one sibling, they are to assign a spokesperson and make decisions together)
- Grandparent
- Grandchild
- Other relatives
- In BC and PEI: A close/trusted friend
- Public Guardian Office (in Ontario, this office is the first in the hierarchy)

You can informally name your SDM but it is wise to formally/ legally name that person. (See Table 2 at the end of this chapter). Strongly consider having these documents drawn up by an estate lawyer if there are any issues of conflict within your family and the possibility someone might contest the validity of the documents.

Difficult situations can arise when frail and elderly spouses are the Substitute Decision Makers.

Joe was 89 and had advanced dementia. He was hospitalized after a bad fall and was not able to go back home. He was no longer capable of choosing his decision makers. His wife Trina was also frail and on her own dementia journey.

Health-care teams discussed Joe's care with Trina but would not discuss it with their two adult daughters because they were under their mother in the hierarchy. The daughters asked for a formal cognitive evaluation of their mother. She was deemed incapable of making decisions and the daughters were then able to make decisions for both of their parents.

2.2 Determine who is best to speak for you

You can choose any capable adult to be your informal SDM. But it's good to think about who this person will be and whether you want them to make decisions for you.

1. In times of stress and difficulty, who provides you with support? Why? (It could be family, friends, neighbours, people you know well from a community group, etc.)

2. If you were unable to direct your own medical care, who would you want to make these decisions for you?

3. Would these people be able to get to you and stay at your side for significant periods of time without it being of undue hardship for them? (For example, would they have to take time off work, fly here to be with you, take time away from their own families?)

4. Can they handle being in hospitals? Can they stay logical (even for brief periods when vital information is being gathered)?

5. Would they be able to speak assertively (not passively and not aggressively) to doctors and nurses?

6. Do you have a back-up person who can help until your loved ones can arrive? Again, this can be a friend or neighbour. Professional health-care navigator-advocates can often fill this role, although they are unable to make decisions for you (see Chapter 1).

2.3 Talk to your Substitute Decision Makers

Your decision makers — whether formal or informal — should know your health-care wishes. If you don't talk to them about what you would want in the event of serious injury, illness, progressing dementia, or at end-of-life, they will have to make decisions for you based on what they know of you and their own values and beliefs. Links to a few uncomfortable, but incredibly important videos in the Resources section available on the download kit included with this book.

Having conversations with the people who might need to speak for you, when you can't speak for yourself, prevents untold amounts of pain and suffering. This is a tough conversation for most people. Chapter 11 will give you a number of ways to start these conversations.

I have seen doctors beg families for guidance when they are trying to decide whether they should proceed with invasive care (examples: putting the patient on a ventilator, doing CPR, starting dialysis, starting artificial feeding or removing feeding tubes) when the procedures may cause more harm than benefit. "Are you sure he never said anything about what he wanted the end of his life to look like?"

Adults will often say they want quality of life over quantity of life, but without guidance, families will often choose quantity over quality.

Health-care professionals want you to discuss your values, beliefs, and preferences for future health care with your loved ones and SDMs.

2.4 When your Substitute Decision Makers can step in to make decisions

You are considered capable or competent to make your own health-care decisions unless deemed incapable or incompetent by a physician or lawyer or another trained professional.

Reasons you may be deemed incapable or incompetent, temporarily or permanently:

a. Being unconscious or in a coma.

b. Receiving large doses of medication that alter your decision-making capability.

c. Having an advanced neurological disease or brain cancer.

d. Moderate to advanced dementia where a trained social worker, physician specialist (usually a geriatrician or a geriatric psychiatrist) or a trained lawyer has determined through testing that the adult is no longer capable. If you are concerned about a loved one's ability to make their own decisions, ask that a formal evaluation be done.

If you are incapable of making your own health-care decisions, your Substitute Decision Maker (SDM) will be asked to make decisions for you.

Michelle was 38 years old when she was diagnosed with aggressive stage three cancer. At that point, her husband, Rob, was travelling for work frequently and she needed a back-up. She went to an estate lawyer and had her husband and her sister, Terri, named co-decision makers, allowing either of them to make decisions independently of each other until the other arrived and then they were to make decisions together.

At the age of 45, her cancer returned and it had metastasized to her brain. Rob and Terri had both had long discussions with Michelle about her end-of-life wishes. Within months her ability to make her own decisions was impaired. Rob was grateful to have Terri at his side to help him make difficult decisions.

3. Write a Formal Substitute Decision Maker Document (at Any Age)

Choosing a legal SDM can be done for free and the documentation is usually simple to understand and prepare (see Resources). It is a document that can alleviate stress for you and your loved ones and it shows the health-care system you've taken the time to make this important decision.

Write up a formal Substitute Decision Maker document if you—

- want to ensure your substitute decision makers can legally make decisions about your living situation, your personal needs, or end-of-life decisions;

- want a close friend or loved one, who is otherwise low on the SDM Hierarchy, to make decisions for you. This is especially important for common-law spouses who may not have met the time guidelines under the provincial rules — or for those with a partner they do not live with;

- do not want a spouse, adult child, or sibling to make health-care decisions for you because of the following:

  - You want your spouse, adult children, or siblings to simply be a loved one, at your side, holding your hand rather than gathering information and making tough decisions.

  - They've got their own health or aging issues.

  - They're not good in stressful medical situations.

  - Their values and beliefs don't align with yours.

  - You're not sure they will honour your wishes.

  - You don't get along with them — or they don't get along with each other;

- need to choose someone nearby as your children, parents, or other relatives are a long way away and it will take time and money to be at your side; or

- have more than one adult child, parent, or sibling who don't get along, and you want or need to assign one of them to make final decisions.

3.1 Formal Substitute Decision Makers by province

There are general guidelines for formal Substitute Decision Makers for all provinces.

The term "Substitute Decision Makers" become the Canada/ North American-wide name for the person has selected, either informally or informally. Every province has a different term for formal Substitute Decision Makers, so we will use the term SDM for clarity.

- Your Substitute Decision Maker is to attempt to check with you prior to making any decisions about your health care.

- Your Substitute Decision Maker cannot —

  - make decisions prohibited by law,

  - ask for Medical Assistance in Dying on your behalf,

  - delegate the role to another person, or

  - authorize treatments not medically necessary including tissue, sterilization, or organ/tissue donation unless stated otherwise in your directive.

4. Reasons to Consult an Estate or Elder-Law Lawyer

There are many reasons to do this kind of document with a lawyer. Some of the major considerations a lawyer could help you document include when you want more than one person to make your future health-care decisions. You may want them to be able to act together or to be able to act independently. Common scenarios include:

- An aging spouse who still wants to make decisions but needs the support and advice from someone else (most commonly an adult child).

- Where distance makes it necessary for one person to begin to make the decisions before another decision maker can be present.

- You want to make sure your loved ones agree about your care options and no one is left out.

There are also future estate issues that may complicate your future care. Unfortunately, it is common that an adult child might not act in your best interest if there is an inheritance waiting for them when you die.

Perhaps you don't want one of your adult children, a sibling, or a relative making decisions for you and you are concerned about the legal repercussions of that decision.

When consulting an estate or elder-law lawyer, ask that all documents — legal SDM form; enduring power of attorney for legal and finances; and an Advance Directive — all be in separate documents so that each of them can be updated separately, as needed.

Table 2

Legal Substitute Decision Maker by Province

Province	Name of SDM	Age and Requirements
British Columbia	Representative	19 and capable; can't be a paid caregiver unless a spouse or an adult child.
Alberta	Agent	18 and capable
Saskatchewan	Proxy	18 and capable
Manitoba	Proxy	18 and capable
Ontario	Attorneys	16, available, willing, and capable of making care decisions. Can't be a paid caregiver unless a spouse or relative.
New Brunswick	Advance Health Directive = Proxy; Power of Attorney = Donee	19 and capable (spouse of any age)
Newfoundland and Labrador	Substitute Decision Maker	19, available, willing, and capable of making care decisions
Nova Scotia	Delegate	19 and capable (spouse of any age)
Prince Edward Island	Proxy or Substitute Decision Maker	16, capable, with knowledge of the situation
Nunavut	Agent	19, available, willing, and capable of making care decisions
Northwest Territories	Agent	19, available, willing, and capable of making care decisions
Yukon	Guardian, Proxy, or Substitute Decision Maker	19, capable, willing, and available

5. Where You Should Keep SDM Documents

Put a copy of any important documents on your fridge with all your other In Case of Emergency documents. Put the original somewhere safe but easy for your SDM to find.

Let your SDMs know what the documents are for and when they might need them.

Give copies to your physicians — your GP and specialists.

Jerry was 63 years old when ALS suddenly took away his ability to make his own health-care and end-of-life wishes. His niece, Teresa stepped in as his formal SDM. Teresa was able to put palliative care in place and she notified the trust company to take over his financial affairs. He had previously been assessed and qualified for Medical Assistance in Dying. While he was no longer capable of making his health-care decisions, he did meet the qualifications process for an advance request, and MAiD was administered. (See Chapter 12 for more information about this topic.)

EIGHT

Determine Your Values, Beliefs, and Preferences for Future Care

When I was a surgical nurse, I looked after Kevin for six months as he battled throat cancer. I liked to get to know my patients but I hadn't gotten to know Kevin at all. I was with him on his last night of life. He was scared and I didn't know how to comfort him. His only son was thousands of miles away and I couldn't reach him. When Kevin died, I was responsible for gathering his belongings. There was so little there. I learned nothing more about him.

We had so many patients spend their last days on our unit, and they often died alone, in a four-bed room. We rarely knew what was important to them in the last days of their lives. I look back on it, and it saddens me. For so many people, things have not changed very much. Too many people die alone in hospitals.

When we let others know what is important to us toward the end of our lives, and at the end of our lives, we can often get a much better death.

Ten years after caring for Kevin, I was a cardiac nurse. Beth was my patient and her heart was coming to a slow, inevitable stop. She was 92 years old and had lived, in her own words, a wonderful life. She had a room full of people with her, and her goddaughter, an opera singer, sang "Amazing Grace" as her heart finally stopped. There was not a dry eye on the ward. Now, in my opinion, that's the way to go.

My mother and I were with my father as he took his last breaths. Afterward, we had tea and biscuits and chatted as if he were there. Just over a year later, my brother and I were with our mother for several days in her hospice room, sleeping beside her at night; she was never alone. Afterward, I helped bathe her. The goodbyes that day were important for us.

Being with both of my parents and performing ceremonies, however simple, was a gift.

The end of your life is important. Be an active part of the journey.

Whether your journey or that of a loved one, find a beautiful journal to write down your thoughts.

1. Think about Your Values and Beliefs

Here are a few examples of what the term "values and beliefs" means (there are no right or wrong answers):

- **I value** my independence; my right to make my own health-care decisions; my family and having them with me at the end of my life; sharing food with those I love; fresh air and nature; my faith in God; my faith in science and medicine.

- **I believe** in my life continuing at all costs (quantity over quality); or, in quality of life over quantity; that my doctors know best and I will trust their judgement; that I know what I want for my future self.

  Sometimes, it is easiest to begin self-reflection by thinking about what we *don't* want our lives to look like.

- **I fear** losing my independence and becoming dependent on others; losing my memories; not being a contributing member of my community; losing control of my bodily functions;

not recognizing my loved ones; my family or health-care team giving up on me. (Often, it's easiest to begin self-reflection by thinking about the way we don't want our lives to look like. Your fears don't have to be rational and they can be contradictory. Fears are our important emotional responses that need to be looked at to be made sense of.)

Our values and beliefs can change with our preferences for future health care as our health becomes more fragile and our options more limited. Often, what is important changes. Our world and our needs get smaller and we are very happy with that.

If your health is declining, you may want to rewrite your advance directive to reflect the changes in what is important to you.

We'll get to your specific preferences for future health care in Chapter 10 on advance directives. In the meantime, fill out Sample 2 (also available on the downloadable forms kit). It will help you sort out your values and beliefs.

My dear friends, Michelle and Reena, founders of Willow have put together an in-depth online toolkit of blogs, and resources, many of them free. For those of you who live or can get to Vancouver, I highly recommend their workshops: willoweol.com/about/

Sample 2
Determine Your Values, Beliefs, and Fears

Rate how important the following are to me	Very Important 4	3	2	Not Important 1
Quality of life over quantity				
Living as long as possible, regardless of quality				
My spiritual beliefs and traditions				
Independence, autonomy, control				
Being mentally alert and competent				
Quality time with family and friends				
Time in nature (fresh air and sunlight)				
My work or volunteering				
Time with my pets				
Care that meets my needs, no matter the cost				
Watching my favourite TV shows and movies				
Birthdays and celebrations				
Preparing, eating and sharing food				
Playing or listening to music				
Vacations/travel				
Writing: Keeping a journal or writing letters				
My hobbies or reading				
Quiet time and/or time to myself				

Other things that are important to me:

_____

_____

_____

Which of the following concern you / do you fear most near the end of life?	Very Important 4	3	2	Not Important 1
Losing control over my own decisions				
Losing my mobility				
Being in uncontrollable pain				
Lingering rather than dying more quickly				
Being incontinent				
Being alone				
Losing the ability to think, being confused most of the time				
Being a burden on loved ones				
Being dependent on others for everyday activities like eating and bathing				
Losing my sight or hearing				

Other things that I fear:

_____

_____

_____

If you could plan them today, imagine what the last days of your life would be like:

☐ Where would I be? _____

_____

☐ What would I be doing? _____

_____

☐ Who would be with me? _____

_____

☐ What would I eat or drink? _____

_____

☐ The comfort of spiritual support from a member of the clergy or someone who shares my religious beliefs: _____

_____

☐ The people who I would want to write a letter or record an audio or video message, perhaps to be read, heard, or watched in the future: _____

_____

☐ How do I want to be remembered? If I were to write my own obituary or epitaph, what would it say? _____

_____

_____

It's time to pause and put this all together. (Consider finding a beautiful journal to write all the following down).

Write out what I want the last days of my life to look like:

_____

_____

_____

Write out how you want to be remembered and what your eulogy or obituary might say. This might be in the form of journal — or having someone record your stories and then having stories transcribed.

Examples: Where I was born; where I have lived; major life moments; things of which I'm most proud.

_____

_____

_____

_____

_____

NINE

Determine Where You Are in Your Health Journey

What is the state of your health? It sounds like a simple question, but one most of us can't always answer accurately. Most of us think we are healthier than we are because change often comes on slowly, and we adapt.

Our doctors often do not tell us the whole story about our health because they feel we won't understand the information, or they are trying to protect us. For example, patients are told something like this: "Your kidneys are not functioning quite as they should. We'll keep an eye on that." That doesn't tell you what level of kidney function you have but it's often easier not to ask further questions. We assume that the doctor will tell us if it's something to worry about.

But, if your doctor has raised some concerns about anything regarding your health, ask more questions and educate yourself on treatments and prognosis. Some health issues seem minor because you feel you are managing them well with medical treatments. But health issues can worsen over time. When you are dealing with more than one issue, it is called a "comorbidity" and that is more concerning for your long-term health and prognosis.

The following workbook shown in Sample 3 is one I've written in conjunction with Dying with Dignity Canada and it is used with permission. It is our hope that this will help you and your loved ones learn and speak the language of the health-care system so you are better prepared for its fast-pace and jargon-filled conversations.

It is our hope that conversations take place prior to crises. Chapter 11 delves deeper into these vital conversations.

Sample 3
Determine the Stages of Life and Health

You're younger than the age of 65 and in good health and fitness

Serious illness and injury can happen at any age. You likely will want any and all treatment for conditions that develop but it's not too early to think about what your values, beliefs, and preferences for care would be if you were in a serious accident, you had a major stroke, or developed any other condition that might render you incapable of speaking for yourself.

No matter your age, who would you want to speak for you? Would they know what you want and how you would not want to live? It's time to start having these conversations and asking yourself these questions. The earlier we have these conversations with our loved ones, the more normal and the less scary the topic is.

At any age, if you have one or more CHRONIC conditions

Once you have more than one chronic condition (controlled or uncontrolled) or any organ failure, no matter how mild, seriously consider thinking and talking about your values, beliefs, and preferences for care.

The most common chronic health conditions are:
- Diabetes (insulin dependent or non-insulin dependent) — even if well controlled.
- High blood pressure (hypertension) — even if well controlled.
- Organ disease:
  - Kidney disease (your doctor may or may not use the word "failure")
  - Heart disease which may include any of the following: angina, heart attack (myocardial infarction), congestive heart failure (CHF), cardiomyopathy (heart enlargement)
  - Lung disease (COPD or other)
  - Liver disease
- Neurological Diseases such as Parkinson's, ALS, Huntington's, Multiple Sclerosis, etc.
- Vascular disease
- Autoimmune disease
- Early to moderate dementia

At any age you have a life-threatening illness (your life-expectancy is less than 1 to 2 years)
This is the stage where many adults wait for their doctors to tell them that things are serious and life-threatening. Patients are scared to bring up their prognosis for several complicated, personal reasons. *But, waiting for your doctors to bring up your mortality can mean waiting too long.* Think about doing your Advance Care Planning early in your diagnosis so it's done and then revisit and revise your Advance Directive as your health changes.

You're older than the age of 65 and relatively healthy
Your body is getting older, a little less resilient, and progressively more fragile. As we age, it's important to think a little deeper and a little more often about what we do and don't want should we become seriously ill or injured. And, it becomes more important to talk to our future health decision-makers about what we want so they are not blindsided by sudden health changes and decisions they may have to make. Put your thoughts to paper and give that to your decision-makers and your clinicians.

You're older than 65 and you are having trouble managing your day-to-day affairs and the activities of daily living. This is referred to as a "frail elder"

We all age differently. It's not the number that counts, but how we are managing with our lives and our health. If you need help with your day-to-day affairs and, especially if you have more than one chronic health condition, you are considered a "frail elder." For a person in this condition, having an Advance Directive — and thinking about Advance Care Planning in general — is imperative.

You're older than 75 — no matter your state of health

This is considered the age where everyone, no matter their apparent health, is more vulnerable and less resilient to disease and injury. *Advance Care Planning should be an urgent call to action at this point in your life.*

Frail elders

We all age differently. Some people in their 50s are frailer than some people in their 90s. The medical system has arbitrarily decided that "frail elders" as 65 and older when in reality people may need supports at an earlier age.

For elderly people, living with chronic conditions can resemble walking at the edge of a cliff. The slightest blow — such as a cold or the flu — will stress their already fragile systems and might push them over the edge. Very often, the health-care system will label this final blow the cause of death, when the cause was more accurately the cumulative effect of illnesses or frailty. *Living Well at the End of Life: Adapting Health Care to Serious Chronic Illness in Old Age,* Joanne Lynn, David M. Adamson, RAND White Paper.

Frailty is associated with several factors which may be reversible or preventable to improve or delay serious outcomes:

- Advancing age
- Vulnerability: poverty and/or isolation
- A decline in the ability to function on your own or to be active
- Poor nutrition or weight loss (Sometimes called "failure to thrive")
- Taking several medications (polypharmacy)
- More than one medical and/or mental health issue, including dementia
- Falls

People are considered frail when they have multiple interacting health problems that are often made worse by social vulnerability (food insecurity, income that is inadequate for need, inadequate shelter, not feeling safe in one's environment, or feeling lonely).

The merit for self-assessment is a basic understanding of where a person might fit on the Clinical Frailty Scale. After that, the final determination requires a CGA (Comprehensive Geriatric Assessment), or other frailty assessment to be done. This then allows you to know which elements might be made better in some way. *In short, the Clinical Frailty Scale [as shown on the next page, with thanks to Dr. Kenneth Rockwood for permission] should be the beginning of an evaluation, and not the end of it.*

Clinical Frailty Scale*

1 **Very Fit** – People who are robust, active, energetic and motivated. These people commonly exercise regularly. They are among the fittest for their age.

2 **Well** – People who have **no active disease symptoms** but are less fit than category 1. Often, they exercise or are very **active occasionally**, e.g. seasonally.

3 **Managing Well** – People whose **medical problems are well controlled**, but are **not regularly active** beyond routine walking.

4 **Vulnerable** – While **not dependent** on others for daily help, often **symptoms limit activities**. A common complaint is being "slowed up", and/or being tired during the day.

5 **Mildly Frail** – These people often have **more evident slowing**, and need help in **high order IADLs** (finances, transportation, heavy housework, medications). Typically, mild frailty progressively impairs shopping and walking outside alone, meal preparation and housework.

6 **Moderately Frail** – People need help with **all outside activities** and with **keeping house**. Inside, they often have problems with stairs and need **help with bathing** and might need minimal assistance (cuing, standby) with dressing.

7 **Severely Frail** – Completely dependent for **personal care**, from whatever cause (physical or cognitive). Even so, they seem stable and not at high risk of dying (within ~ 6 months).

8 **Very Severely Frail** – Completely dependent, approaching the end of life. Typically, they could not recover even from a minor illness.

9. **Terminally Ill** - Approaching the end of life. This category applies to people with a **life expectancy <6 months**, who are **not otherwise evidently frail**.

Scoring frailty in people with dementia

The degree of frailty corresponds to the degree of dementia. Common **symptoms in mild dementia** include forgetting the details of a recent event, though still remembering the event itself, repeating the same question/story and social withdrawal.

In **moderate dementia**, recent memory is very impaired, even though they seemingly can remember their past life events well. They can do personal care with prompting.

In **severe dementia**, they cannot do personal care without help.

* 1. Canadian Study on Health & Aging. Revised 2008.
2. K. Rockwood et al. A global clinical measure of fitness and frailty in elderly people. CMAJ 2005;173:489-495.

© 2009. Version 1.2_EN. All rights reserved. Geriatric Medicine Research, Dalhousie University, Halifax, Canada. Permission granted to copy for research and educational purposes only.

DALHOUSIE UNIVERSITY
Inspiring Minds

Clinical Frailty Scale: Used with permission from Geriatric Medicine Research, Dalhousie University: https://www.dal.ca/sites/gmr/our-tools/clinical-frailty-scale.html

Frailty in Older Adults, Early Identification and Management

It's time to pause and do some homework. After an honest assessment, where are you in your health journey? If you don't know, it's time to ask your physicians or nurse practitioners for their honest assessment, and more testing and more referrals, if needed.

Write down where you are in your life health journey, based on what you determined, above.

_____

_____

_____

_____

_____

_____

_____

TEN

Advance Directives: Considering and Writing Your Wishes for Future Care

An advance directive is part of the process of advance care planning. An advance directive is a document outlining your written wishes for future health care if you cannot speak for yourself. In most provinces, it is a legally binding document that must be followed by your health-care team and your Substitute Decision Makers. It must apply directly to your health care. It is only in place while you are still alive.

Advance directive is the term commonly used for a legal health-care document around the world. However, each province set up their own health-care legislation 20 to 30 years ago, and each uses slightly different terms. We are using the term "advance directive" for clarity and simplicity. Table 3 shows the terms for each province.

A written document is not required if you have told those who may need to speak for you about your wishes for future health care. But there are a lot of things that can go sideways by relying on conversations alone:

Table 3
Advance Directive Terms by Province

	Age Directive Can Be Put in Place	What the Directive Is Called
British Columbia	19 and capable	Advance Directive
Alberta	18 and capable	Personal Directive
Saskatchewan	16 and capable	Health Care Directive
Manitoba	16 and capable	Health Care Directive
Ontario	16 and capable and has a genuine concern for health of represented party	Power of Attorney for Personal Care
New Brunswick	19 and capable	Advance Health Directive
Newfoundland and Labrador	16 and capable	Advance Health Directive
Nova Scotia	19 and capable and willing to make decisions.	Personal Directive
Prince Edward Island	16 and capable and available.	Health Care Directive
Northwest Territories	19 and understand the nature and effect of Personal Directive	Personal Directive
Nunavut	19 and understand the nature and effect of Personal Directive	Personal Directive
Yukon	16 and capable	Directive

- We feel we can't have conversations with those we love.

- The people who know what we want might not be available in a time of crisis. Emergency health-care treatments will proceed until they can be contacted.

- Or, they might panic, and will ask for health-care treatments (such as resuscitation), even though that is something you have decided you don't want.

This chapter will go through the process of determining where you are in your health journey, determining your values and beliefs, and then writing your advance directive.

1. A Quick Review of the Difference between Advance Care Planning and Estate Planning

Advance care planning and estate planning are often done at the same time. Advance care planning includes conversations and documentation (health, personal planning, and financial planning) that can be put in force while you are still alive. Estate planning (your will and naming of executor, and life insurance) is legal documentation about your estate and is only put in force after your death. See Figure 2.

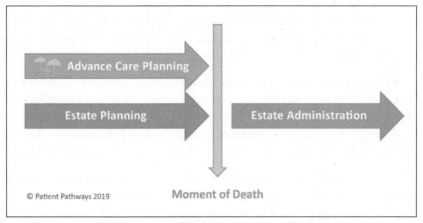

Figure 1: Moment of Death in Relation to Care Planning

Advance Care Planning is the following:

1. Financial Documentation: Enduring Powers of Attorney (Chapter 5).

2. Determine who will speak for you if you can't speak for yourself — Substitute Decision Makers (SDM) — and assigning them informally or formally. (Chapter 7).

3. Determine your values and beliefs and your wishes for future health care (Chapter 8).

4. Determine where you are in your health journey (Chapter 9).

5. Writing an advance directive and other supporting documents such as a request or order for No CPR/DNR/Resucitation.

6. Talk about your values, wishes and preferences for future care to your loved ones, your SDMs, and your health-care team. (Chapter 11).

7. Considerations for the end of your life (Chapter 12).

The pinnacle of empowerment is looking at, and planning for, what you want your life to look like as you approach end of life. And, realizing that serious injury and illness can happen at any time, to anyone, at any age.

As much as 93 percent of Canadians think it's important to communicate their wishes for future care should they become seriously ill but only 36 percent have actually done so. (To die well, we must talk about death before the end of life: Tamara Sussman; The Conversation: https://theconversation.com/to-die-well-we-must-talk-about-death-before-the-end-of-life-124256.)

Throughout the advance care planning communities — and there are a lot of us having these discussions — we're trying to get you to have these discussions, too. Many of us use the quote, "It seems too early until it's too late," because as health-care providers we know, through experience, we simply don't know when "too late" will be.

If you were able to go into an emergency room or an intensive care unit and talk to patients and families, every one of them would say, "I could never have imagined this. He was walking and talking this morning, just leading his life and now it will never be the same." Thinking that this won't happen to you or someone you love is being intentionally naive. Looking at the possibility of serious illness and planning for it doesn't take away hope — but it can prevent unnecessary emotional suffering.

Like sex education, not talking about sex might get you pregnant — and not talking about death might result in receiving health-care treatments you don't want or that will do more harm than good. The earlier you start thinking and talking about your values and beliefs, and thinking about your preferences for future care, the easier the conversations become.

"Death is part of life. While death is inevitable, a bad death is not." (Dr. Perez Protto, Medical director, End of Life Center, Cleveland Clinic.)

2. What Is an Advance Directive?

Every province has a different name for an advance directive and the breakdown of the names of documents is provided in Table 3. There are so many different terms to describe a health directive: an advance care plan, a living will, or just the inaccurate word, "directive." Gradually, advance directive is becoming the term that most health-care professionals, lawyers, and notaries are using across North America, and the term we will use here.

Having an advance directive means you have put your future wishes for health care into writing. It must directly apply to your health-care wishes. It should be clear, short, and instantly interpretable to medical orders. In most provinces (except Ontario), an advance directive is a legally binding document.

An advance directive is a written document, signed, dated, and witnessed, that lets your loved ones and your health-care team know what you do and do not want your life to look like should you be seriously injured, be seriously ill (likely a temporary state), or in a state of cognitive decline when you can no longer speak for yourself due to a neurological disease or dementia (likely a permanent state).

3. Understanding Resuscitation and "No CPR"

Before moving forward, understanding cardiopulmonary resuscitation (CPR) is a first step. Whether it is wanted is the first question loved ones will be asked in a life-threatening situation in the community by bystanders, first responders and paramedics, and emergency room and hospital staff.

Most people who go into cardiac arrest or have a lethal (life-ending) heart rhythm, will have this occur at home, or while out and about in the community [Sudden Cardiac Death (sudden cardiac arrest): Cleveland Clinic: https://my.clevelandclinic.org/health/diseases/17522-sudden-cardiac-death-sudden-cardiac-arrest]. It is vital to think about whether you want to be resuscitated and what you need to do if you've decided you don't want CPR and resuscitation started. You won't be able to speak for yourself so you must have appropriate documentation immediately available so the trained health-care teams know your wishes.

Should you decide not to have CPR, your decision needs to be clearly written at the top of your Advance Directive, and in some provinces, a formal health-care order must be signed. It is also recommended that you get a medical alert bracelet — because your decision not to have CPR is only as good as the ability to let the trained public, first responders, paramedics, and emergency room personnel know your wishes.

In several provinces, the only way to ensure you do not have CPR in your home or in the community is to have a "No CPR or DNR" form signed by your doctor. A medical alert bracelet is highly advised!

The medical community is aware that your chances of surviving — and certainly thriving — after a cardiac arrest are low. But the public's understanding of the what happens during and after cardiac arrest, and what your life will look like if you survive, is unrealistic, and likely harmful.

It's important to look deeply at the possibility of CPR and what you want to look like if you survive. If you choose to have CPR, everything will be done to save you, including being in ICU, on a ventilator. Your advance directive should state when you would want life-support evaluated and, possibly, discontinued.

Choosing not to have CPR does not mean that everything else won't be done. We have put together a very comprehensive list in the information below so you can choose the level of treatment you want performed.

Finally, if you decide you don't want CPR performed, it is extremely important you discuss your decision with your loved ones, your substitute decision makers, and anyone who cares for you, so your wishes are honoured if you have a cardiac arrest. Anyone who is with you is likely to panic and ask that CPR is performed, and your conversation prior to an emergency will make it easier. See Chapter 11 on vital conversations with those you love and those who care for you.

In hospital, it is up to you and/or your substitute decision makers to start a discussion with your health-care team about your decision about not having CPR — and whether that decision applies in hospital, or whether your medical directive and medical levels of care orders should be modified for surgeries or treatment.

CPR means Cardio-Pulmonary Resuscitation: "Cardio" means heart; "pulmonary" means lungs; "resuscitation" means to try and restart a person's heartbeat and breathing when they stop. CPR is the act of manual, aggressive compressions on your chest.

"No CPR" is the same as "Do Not Resuscitate" or DNR.

In British Columbia, the legal term for a request not to resuscitate is "No CPR" (No Chest Compressions) and in the rest of the provinces it is "DNR (Do Not Resuscitate)."

CPR is not what most people think it is: It is not a decision that should be taken lightly and the consequences of being resuscitated are serious. If you survive, at the very least, your sternum and ribs will be broken. You will be on a ventilator for an undetermined length of time, increasing your chances of life-threatening infections.

Think about life sustaining treatment:

- In what stage of life are you?

- Do you want quality of life, or quantity?

Should everyone have CPR? No, but CPR can work for adults who are reasonably healthy. CPR is most effective when initiated immediately after cardiac arrest.

But, CPR is usually not effective for adults with medical conditions with damage to their heart, lungs, kidneys, and brain, or adults who are at the natural end of their lives.

Studies have shown the chances of survival with CPR depend on the health of the patient. In the overall population younger than the age of 75, 82 out of 100 will die; 18 will survive CPR and leave the hospital. For people with serious illnesses such as cancer, heart, or kidney disease, 90 out of 100 will die; 10 will survive CPR (but might not leave hospital). For people who have critical illnesses and are in the intensive care unit, 98 out of 100 will die; 2 will survive CPR (but might not leave hospital). For the overall population older than the age of 75, 85 out of 100 will die; 15 will survive CPR (but might not leave hospital). (Living Well, Planning Well: An Advance Care Planning Resource for Lawyers: www.advancecareplanning.ca/resource/living-well-planning-well-lawyers-resource, accessed January, 2020.)

4. Understanding Hospital Medical Orders of Levels of Care

Until recently, if CPR and resuscitation were not wanted or were seen as futile, doctors would simply write an order that said, "No CPR" or "DNR." That often left medical and nursing teams confused. They wondered if they were just providing comfort care — or were they to do everything up to, but not including CPR? There were too many shades of grey.

Over the last several years, most provinces have introduced medical orders that are to be put at the front of all hospitalized patients' charts. For patients who are seriously ill or injured, health-care providers are to ask each patient or Substitute Decision Makers (SDMs)

Table 4
No CPR/DNR Forms by Province

	No CPR or DNR forms
British Columbia	No CPR form (required if cardiac arrest occurs at home or in community): https://www2.gov.bc.ca/assets/gov/health/forms/302fil.pdf
Alberta	Goals of Care Designation (GCD) Order This form is completed in the presence of your doctor and kept on file. https://www.albertahealthservices.ca/frm-103547.pdf
Saskatchewan	No specific form. Wishes for No CPR or DNR are to be written on your advance directive or on medical orders of **Goals of Care**. See more at: https://www.saskatoonhealthregion.ca/patients/Pages/Resuscitation-Plan.aspx
Manitoba	No specific form. Wishes for No CPR or DNR are to be written on your health-care directive.
Ontario	DNR form: http://www.forms.ssb.gov.on.ca/mbs/ssb/forms/ssbforms.nsf/FormDetail?OpenForm&ENV=WWE&NO=014-4519-45
New Brunswick	As written on **Advance Health Care Directive Form**: https://www2.gnb.ca/content/gnb/en/departments/health/patientinformation/content/advance_health_care_directives.html
Newfoundland and Labrador	Talk to your doctor. No form available.
Nova Scotia	DNR form: Does not have to be signed by physician: https://novascotia.ca/dhw/publications/PFEDH_DNR_form.pdf
Prince Edward Island	No specific form. Wishes for No CPR or DNR are to be written on your health-care directive.
Northwest Territories	No specific form. Wishes for No CPR or DNR are to be written on your personal directive.
Nunavut	No form. Wishes for No CPR or DNR are to be written on your personal directive.
Yukon	Resuscitation and Care http://www.yukon.ca/en/resucitation-and-care

if the patient has expressed or documented wishes about future care through an advance directive and/or representation agreement.

"No CPR/DNR/No Chest Compression" orders will automatically be suspended for surgery and other procedures involving anesthesia or procedural sedation and treatment will be provided at the discretion of the Most Responsible Physician Provider. If you do not want resuscitation during surgery, you must take the initiative to speak directly with your surgeon and anesthetist.

Except in extreme circumstances (when you are in a critical situation) and only when you and your Substitute Decision Maker cannot be consulted, medical levels of care orders should be reviewed upon every admission.

In most circumstances, if physician specialists and surgeons deem the patient to be reasonably healthy and the procedure/surgery to be uncomplicated, the doctor can sign the medical levels of care orders without having a discussion with you.

Your Most Responsible Provider (MRP — physician or nurse practitioner) has the ultimate choice in not initiating (or removing) care or treatment based on "Expectations of Care Not Considered Beneficial." If you or your loved one is in a critical health situation, it is important to know that there are likely specific policies in place that allow a physician to override the wishes of the patient or family, if it is unlikely that efforts will be futile. (The Challenge of Futile Treatment: Journal of Medical Ethics, July 2016.)

This is an example from Vancouver Coastal Health in BC:

"It is the responsibility of the Physician/Health Care Team to determine the most appropriate care to offer to the patient/client/resident (patient), based on the best interests of the patient and informed by what the patient wants or would have wanted if the patient is not able to speak for himself or herself, as communicated by a representative of the patient, ideally through an advance care planning document.

"There will be situations in which the Physician/Team decides not to offer, or decides not to continue to offer, care that the patient or his/her representative wants/demands, such as cardiopulmonary resuscitation, mechanical ventilation, food and fluids by artificial means, etc.

"There is no obligation to offer care simply because it is requested, however expectations for (continued) care that the Team does not consider appropriate must be addressed respectfully."

– VCH Risk Management, revised February 2014

5. Level of Care – Glossary of Terms

Before you write your advance directive, it's a good idea to get familiar with some terms.

Table 5
In-Hospital Levels of Care Documents by Province

To be discussed and signed by you and physician in hospital.

British Columbia	**MOST – Medical Orders for Scope of Treatment:** Vancouver Coastal Health; Island Health; Interior Health; & Northern Health **Options for Care:** Providence Health
Alberta	**Goals of Care:** https://www.albertahealthservices.ca/info/Page9099.aspx
Saskatchewan	**Advance Care Planning: Goals of Care Guides** – Reference Chart: http://www.rqhealth.ca/sla-physicians-news/advance-care-planning-goals-of-care-guides
Manitoba	**Advance Care Planning Goals of Care** https://www.wrha.mb.ca/acp/files/professionals/Workbook.pdf
Ontario	**Advance Care Planning Goals of Care Designation** http://extcontent.covenanthealth.ca/Policy/vii-b-350.pdf
New Brunswick	Goals of Care not instituted at time of writing.
Newfoundland and Labrador	Goals of Care not instituted at time of writing.
Nova Scotia	Goals of Care not instituted at time of writing.
Prince Edward Island	**Goals of Care:** https://www.princeedwardisland.ca/sites/default/files/forms/goals_of_care_form.pdf
Nunavut	Goals of Care not instituted at time of writing.
Northwest Territories	Goals of Care not instituted at time of writing.
Yukon	Goals of Care not instituted at time of writing.

Artificial hydration: The use of intravenous fluids (IV) to maintain hydration (fluid balance) and to deliver medications, most commonly antibiotics. At end-of-life, these fluids can prolong life and discussions should take place with you (if you are still capable), health-care professionals, and your substitute decision makers.

Artificial nutrition: Also called enteral feeding, is liquid nutrition delivering carbohydrates, fats, protein, and vitamins via a nasogastric tube (a tube in the nose, down to the stomach), and into the stomach; or, when nutrition is needed long term, via a surgically inserted tube through the abdominal wall and into the top of the small bowel (bypassing the stomach). Risks versus benefit of these treatments should be reviewed with a discussion of short-term versus long-term nutrition therapy.

Defibrillation: A series of electrical shocks on the chest to reset the heart's rhythm. Often there are non-life-threatening rhythms such as atrial fibrillation that are easily corrected by defibrillation. Discussions with your physician before refusing defibrillation are recommended. You may want to add comments to your advance directive regarding when you would want attempts at defibrillation discontinued.

Dialysis: A process where a machine filters waste from your blood — a function normally performed by your kidneys. Often our kidneys take a "hit" and go into shock in an acute medical event, especially after a heart attack, cardiac arrest, or major surgery. Dialysis can take over while the kidneys rest and recover. However, if you already have some kidney failure, before a serious health event, your kidneys will take a further assault and may not recover. Ongoing dialysis for months or years is a decision that should not be taken lightly, and this should be discussed at length by you and/or your substitute decision makers with your health-care team. If you choose to have dialysis on your advance directive, you may want to add comments about when you would want it discontinued.

Intensive Care and Critical Care Units (ICU and CCU): The names of the units are used interchangeably. The units have more nurses and doctors per patient, and there is monitoring and life-support equipment and treatments including ventilators and dialysis.

Palliative Care — Oxygen for comfort: Oxygen does not prolong life but can making breathing easier and less alarming for your loved ones.

Palliative Care — Non-invasive oral suctioning: Some patients at end-of-life are no longer able to swallow and saliva builds up in their mouths. It is a normal part of the dying process, but it can be disturbing to loved ones. With oral suctioning, a tube is put into the mouth and the fluids sucked out. It should be done gently with a rubber-tipped catheter to prevent tissue damage and bleeding.

Palliative Care — Pleasure Feeding: This includes whatever you do want and can eat or drink at the end of your life. It is not recommended for patients who have an impaired swallowing reflex as choking may cause aspiration pneumonia. Be aware that any food or fluid will prolong life. Note that withholding food and fluids can be distressing for loved ones, but the patient's desire and need for food and fluids will naturally diminish or disappear at end-stage and it is a normal process of dying.

Respiratory — Non-invasive respiratory support: Where breathing and oxygen support are provided for acute respiratory failure using a mask or similar device without a tube being put down the throat or via a tracheostomy. This is usually provided by CPAP (continuous positive airway pressure) or BiPAP (Bilevel Positive Airway Pressure).

Respiratory — ventilator: A machine that provides breathing support and oxygen through a tube down the throat via a tube in the mouth or a tracheostomy (surgical incision at the base of the throat). It might be used short-term during or after surgery, but it might also be used long-term for the rest of the person's life. Benefits versus risks should be discussed with the adult or substitute decision makers, based on the patient's values and beliefs.

Surgical procedures might restore previous function or reduce pain: The survival benefit of surgery should be considered together with the patients' goal of care; there is an opportunity to improve quality of care regardless of how the [issue] is managed. The most common surgical procedures in palliative and end-of-life situations is hip-fracture repair.

6. Determine the Appropriate Level of Care

Consider which level of care is most appropriate for you at your age and your state of health. There are additional options under each level of care in order to get even more specific.

Add the level you choose (and applicable sub-categories) to your advance directive.

Note: Prior to writing your advance directive, please talk to your physician or nurse practitioner for full guidance and which level is appropriate to your situation when using the designations in Table 4.

Every province has slightly different levels of care definitions. We have tried to standardize these and turn them into plain language.

7. Write Your Advance Directive

The following are examples of completed advance directives for each level of care. Feel free to use or modify them for your own situation (consult your lawyer).

The following information is required for a legal document.

This is the [Advance] Directive for: [change the name of the document, depending on your province – see Table 3]

Full name

Date of Birth

Health Number

Address

Substitute Decision Makers, relationship [including formal SDM document if applicable – and attach copy] and contact information:

This [Advance] Directive Revokes any previous directives.

These are my values, beliefs, and preferences for health care when I can't speak for myself.

At the end of the Advance Directive:

- Signature and printed name of the adult

- Signature and printed name of the witness(es)

- Address and phone numbers of the witness(es)

The following are examples of phrases that could be in advance directives, for each stage of health.

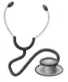

Perform all resuscitation and CPR:

- I understand that all medical intervention including defibrillation, being on a ventilator, and being in a critical care unit will be provided.

- Wherever possible, discuss risks versus benefits of ventilation and ongoing therapy or surgeries with my Substitute Decision Makers, and continue or discontinue care, based on my values and beliefs, below.

- At this point in my life I am not seriously ill. I want to be resuscitated and put on life support if there is a probability that I will recover to some extent. However, after a thorough assessment and waiting period, if I have serious brain damage or there is little or no brain activity, I want life support to be removed as soon as recipients have been found for any organs you can use.

Values and beliefs:

Please consider these as you move forward with treatment decisions:

- Quality of life is more important to me than quantity of life.

- Independence and control of my own life are fundamental.

- I must have a good chance of a full recovery. I am willing to work hard at recovery – but there must be a good chance I will be able to have a full life and live independently.

- If there is a significant chance, I will need supportive care (examples: in ICU, at home, or in residential care) for the rest of my life, I do not want heroic actions taken. Let infections take their course.

- If it is likely I will die, I would like to have my family and loved ones present.

End-of-life wishes:

If possible and reasonable, I would like to die:

- In hospice or palliative care.

I would like the following spiritual ceremonies to be performed before/after my death –

My cultural beliefs are important to me. I would like the following –

Other important information –

Example of "modified resuscitation" not including CPR:

Do not perform CPR but allow transfer to critical care for all treatments, including advanced medications, intravenous antibiotics, and surgeries that are likely to maintain or improve my quality of life.

- Wherever possible, discuss risks versus benefits of any treatments or surgeries with my Substitute Decision Makers, and continue or discontinue treatment, based on my values and beliefs, below.

- Allow a ventilator if it will likely be of benefit over the short-term.

- Allow defibrillation to restart or regulate my heart rhythm

- Allow artificial hydration and nutrition. Please discontinue hydration and feeding if they are not benefiting me and my condition is continuing to decline.

Values and Beliefs:

Please consider these as you move forward with treatment decisions:

- Quality of life is more important to me than quantity of life.

- Independence and control of my own life are fundamental.

- I must have a good chance of a full recovery. I am willing to work hard at recovery – but there must be a good chance I will be able to have a full life and live independently.

- If there is a significant chance, I will need supportive care (examples: in ICU, at home, or in residential care) for the rest of my life, I do not want heroic actions taken. Let infections take their course.

- If it is likely I will die, I would like to have my family and loved ones present.

End-of-life wishes:

If possible and reasonable, I would like to die:

- In hospice or palliative care.

I would like the following spiritual ceremonies to be performed before/after my death –

My cultural beliefs are important to me. I would like the following –

Other important information –

Example of "No CPR/DNR," send to hospital but do not transfer to Critical Care

Do not perform CPR or resuscitation: Comfort Care & Transport to Hospital for higher level of care for treatments, including advanced medications, intravenous antibiotics, and surgeries that are likely to maintain my quality of life.

- Wherever possible, discuss risks versus benefits of any treatments or surgeries with my Substitute Decision Makers, and continue or discontinue care, based on my values and beliefs, below.

(Remember that all of these are options. Change or remove any of the following as needed.)

- Allow non-invasive respiratory support
- Allow surgical procedures in attempt to restore my previous level of function
- Allow CPR and resuscitation during surgery or recovery room only
- Allow short-term stay in critical care for additional support
- Allow short-term ventilation support
- Allow short-term artificial nutrition

Values and beliefs:

Please consider these as you move forward with treatment decisions:

- Quality of life is more important to me than quantity of life.
- Wherever possible, discuss risks versus benefits of any treatments or surgeries with my Substitute Decision Makers, based on my values and beliefs.
- If my condition continues to decline, please discontinue all treatments, surgeries, antibiotics.
- Feed me and allow IV fluids, but do not provide artificial hydration or nutrition (tube feeding).
- Discontinue feeding and IV fluids if they are not showing to have any benefit and my condition is continuing to decline.
- If it is likely I will die, I would like to have my family and loved ones present.

End-of-life wishes:

If possible and reasonable, I would like to die in my home (or current place of residence).

I would like the following spiritual ceremonies to be performed before/after my death –

My cultural beliefs are important to me. I would like the following –

Other important information –

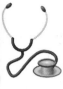

Example of No CPR/DNR; treat me at home/residential care/ palliative care; do not transfer to hospital:

- Do not perform CPR: Comfort Care & Minimal Supportive Care only – Do not transfer to higher level of care (except in exceptional situations – see below). I am nearing the end of my life. I no longer want active medical treatment.

(Remember that all of these are options. Change or remove any of the following as needed.)

- Allow transfer to hospital for surgical procedures for comfort only (example: fractures).
- Allow oral antibiotics for short-term management of infections.
- When I can no longer feed myself: Feed me but do not provide IV fluids or artificial hydration or nutrition (tube feeding). Discontinue feeding if it is not showing to have any benefit and my condition is continuing to decline.

Values and beliefs:

Please consider these as you move forward with treatment decisions:

- Quality of life is more important to me than quantity of life.
- If my condition continues to decline, please discontinue all treatments, surgeries, antibiotics.
- Feed me and allow IV fluids, but do not provide artificial hydration or nutrition (tube feeding).
- Discontinue feeding me if it is not showing to have any benefit and my condition is continuing to decline.
- If it is likely I will die, I would like to have my family and loved ones present.

End-of-life wishes:

- If possible and reasonable, I would like to die in my home (or current place of residence) – or transfer to hospice for pain and symptom management.

I would like the following spiritual ceremonies to be performed before/after my death –

My cultural beliefs are important to me. I would like the following –

Other important information –

Example of "Withdrawal of Treatment" (this can be added to any advance directive):

Withdrawal of treatment: Do not perform CPR: Comfort Care Only: I have an advancing disease or dementia.

When the following occurs, I no longer want medical treatment (antibiotics or other life-extending measures). I am prepared for my life to end when:

- I have unbearable pain.
- I no longer recognize my loved ones.
- I am consistently incontinent of urine or stool.
- When I am dependent on others for all my care needs (examples: eating, toileting, bathing, transferring).

Provide supportive care (pain management and oxygen for comfort).

(Remember that all of these are options. Change or remove any of the following as needed.)

- Stop artificial hydration and nutrition.
- Stop investigations such as blood work and vital sign monitoring.
- Allow non-invasive oral suctioning.
- Allow pleasure feeds (**Note:** this may prolong life).
- Allow oxygen for comfort.

End-of-life wishes:

- If possible and reasonable, I would like to die in my home (or current place of residence) – or transfer to hospice for pain and symptom management.

I would like the following spiritual ceremonies to be performed before/after my death –

My cultural beliefs are important to me. I would like the following –

Other important information –

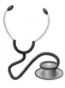

Comfort Care Only:

Do not perform CPR: Comfort Care Only: I am at the natural end of my life. (Remember that all of these are options. Change or remove any of the following as needed.)

- Stop artificial hydration and nutrition.
- Stop investigations such as blood work and vital sign monitoring.
- Allow non-invasive oral suctioning.
- Allow pleasure feeds (**Note:** this may prolong life).
- Allow oxygen for comfort.

End-of-life wishes:

- If possible and reasonable, I would like to die in my home (or current place of residence) – or transfer to hospice for pain and symptom management.

I would like the following spiritual ceremonies to be performed before/after my death –

My cultural beliefs are important to me. I would like the following –

Other important information –

Remember, you can revoke and and write a new advance directive at any time as long as you are still capable. This will be important as personal circumstances and your health changes.

8. Final Steps with Your Advance Directive

For advance care planning and directives resources consult a qualified lawyer and see the Resources section on the download kit. Remember to do the following:

1. Have vital conversations about your decisions with your loved ones and your health-care team (see Chapter 11).

2. When written, sign your advance directive and get it witnessed.

3. Put a copy on the fridge along with any other important ACP documents. (Indicate where the original can be found.)

4. Upload it to a central repository (examples: Nidus.ca in BC or with CARP Health 360, nationally).

5. Give a copy to your substitute decision makers and ask them to have it somewhere handy and to bring it to the hospital, if needed.

6. Have all physicians scan a copy of this and other important ACP documents to your file.

For more information on advance directives and living wills consult *Living Wills Kit*, another Self-Counsel Press title, and your lawyer.

Sample 4
Determine Your Level of Care

As you read the Levels of Care, think about:
- Where are you in your life journey?
- Where do you live?
- Where do you want to die?

Transplantation and transfusions

If you have any beliefs around receiving tissue and/or blood products, add this information to the *top* of your Advance Directive:

- I consent to organ or tissue transplantation   ☐ Yes   ☐ No
- I consent to receiving blood or blood products   ☐ Yes   ☐ No
- I consent to receiving plasma only   ☐ Yes   ☐ No

Perform all resuscitation and CPR:
- Goal is to extend life. I understand that all medical intervention including defibrillation, being on a ventilator, and being in a critical care unit will be provided.
- Wherever possible, discuss risks versus benefits of ventilation and ongoing therapy or surgeries with my Substitute Decision Makers, and continue or discontinue care, based on my values and beliefs, below.

If you want CPR, these are examples of what you might want to add to your Advance Directive:

- **Full CPR and resuscitation:** I am still relatively young. At this point in my life I am not seriously ill. I want to be resuscitated and put on life support if there is a probability that I will recover to some extent. However, after a thorough assessment and waiting period, if I have serious brain damage or there is little or no brain activity, I do not want to be put on life support, or I want it to be removed as soon as recipients have been found for any organs you can use.

  OR

- **Full CPR and resuscitation:** I want to be resuscitated and put on life support with all efforts to keep me alive as long as possible. I will leave it up to my doctors to decide when no further measures can be taken or should be suspended.

Do *not* perform CPR but allow transfer to critical care for all treatments, including advanced medications, intravenous antibiotics and surgeries that are likely to maintain or improve my quality of life. *(See Summary of Medical Definitions above.)*

- Goal is to extend life for *reversible* conditions only.
- Wherever possible, discuss risks versus benefits of any treatments or surgeries with my Substitute Decision Makers, and continue or discontinue treatment, based on my values and beliefs, below.
  - Allow a ventilator   ☐ Yes   ☐ No
  - Allow defibrillation to restart or regulate my heart rhythm   ☐ Yes   ☐ No
  - Allow artificial hydration and nutrition   ☐ Yes   ☐ No

Do not perform CPR: Comfort Care & Transport to Hospital for higher level of care for treatments, including advanced medications, intravenous antibiotics and surgeries that are likely *to maintain* my quality of life.

- Goal is conservative management of medical conditions with specific short-term symptom-directed care to maintain current level of function.
- Wherever possible, discuss risks versus benefits of any treatments or surgeries with my Substitute Decision Makers, and continue or discontinue care, based on my values and beliefs, below.
  - Allow non-invasive respiratory support   ☐ Yes   ☐ No
  - Allow surgical procedures in attempt to restore previous   ☐ Yes   ☐ No
    level of function
  - Allow resuscitation during surgery or recovery room only   ☐ Yes   ☐ No
  - Allow short-term stay in critical care for additional support   ☐ Yes   ☐ No
  - Allow short-term ventilation support   ☐ Yes   ☐ No
  - Allow short-term artificial nutrition   ☐ Yes   ☐ No

Do not perform CPR: Comfort Care & Minimal Supportive Care only – Do *not* transfer to higher level of care (except in exceptional situations – see below).

- Goal is conservative management of medical conditions with specific short-term symptom directed treatment.
- I am nearing the end of my life. I no longer want active medical treatment.
- Wherever possible, discuss risks versus benefits of any treatments or surgeries with my Substitute Decision Makers, base on my values and beliefs.
  - Allow transfer to hospital for surgical procedures for comfort only
    (Example: fractures)   ☐ Yes   ☐ No
  - Allow oral antibiotics for short-term management of infections   ☐ Yes   ☐ No

When I can no longer feed myself
(Add only one)

☐ Feed me *and* provide IV fluids and artificial hydration and nutrition (tube feeding) if deemed appropriate.

     ☐ *(Optional)* Discontinue feeding and artificial nutrition if feeding is not showing any benefit and my condition continues to decline. *(Important for short-term illness, injury or surgery, from which you are likely to recover to some extent.)*

☐ Feed me and *allow* IV fluids, but do *not* provide artificial hydration or nutrition (tube feeding).

     ☐ *(Optional)* Discontinue feeding and IV fluids if they are not showing to have any benefit and my condition is continuing to decline.

☐ Feed me but do *not* provide IV fluids or artificial hydration or nutrition (tube feeding).

     ☐ *(Optional)* Discontinue feeding if it is not showing to have any benefit and my condition is continuing to decline.

☐ Do *not* feed me and do *not* provide intravenous (IV) fluids or any artificial hydration or nutrition. I understand this will lead to my death.

Sample 4 – Continued

Do not perform CPR: Comfort Care Only
Goal is maximizing comfort care and symptom control at the end of life.
- Stop artificial hydration and nutrition
- Stop investigations such as blood work and vital sign monitoring

(Recommended for comfort care:)
- Allow non-invasive oral suctioning   ☐ Yes ☐ No
- Allow pleasure feeds *(Note: this may prolong life)*   ☐ Yes ☐ No
- Allow oxygen for comfort   ☐ Yes ☐ No

Withdrawal of treatment
(Add only if applicable)

☐ I have an advancing disease or dementia. When the following occur, I no longer want medical treatment (antibiotics or other life-extending measures). Provide supportive care (pain management and oxygen for comfort). I am prepared for my life to end *when*:

_____

_____

_____

(Add ALL that are applicable.)

☐ Unbearable pain.

☐ I no longer recognize my loved ones.

☐ I am consistently incontinent of urine or stool.

☐ When I am dependent on others for all my care needs (examples: eating, toileting, bathing, transferring).

Add your Values and Beliefs:
(Choose ALL that are applicable.)

☐ I am willing for anything and everything to be tried to save my life. I am not ready to die.

☐ I trust my health-care team to determine my treatment options.

☐ *Quality* of life is more important to me than *quantity* of life.

☐ Independence and control of my own life are fundamental.

☐ I must have a good chance of a full recovery. I am willing to work hard at recovery – but there must be a good chance I will be able to have a full life and live independently.

☐ If there is a significant chance I will need supportive care (examples: in ICU, at home, or in residential care) for the rest of my life, I do not want heroic actions taken. Let infections take their course.

☐ I would like my body or organs donated.

☐ I am registered organ donor.

☐ If it is likely I will die I would like to have my family and loved ones present.

That spiritual ceremonies be performed before/after my death:

_____

_____

_____

My cultural beliefs are important to me. In my own words:

_____

_____

_____

Other important values and beliefs:

_____

_____

_____

End-of-life wishes

If possible and reasonable, I would like to die:
(Select only one *of these statements)*

☐ At home (if death is reasonably foreseeable, a signed medical form should be attached).

☐ In hospice or palliative care.

☐ In hospital.

At the end of my life it's important to me:

_____

_____

_____

_____

_____

_____

ELEVEN

Vital, Ongoing Conversations with Those You Love and Those Who Will Care for You

This chapter is near the end of the book, because you need to get clear about what is important to you before you begin to talk to your team: your loved ones, those who might have to step in and speak up for you, and those who are providing medical treatment.

Hopefully, you've been having conversations with your team throughout this journey. But, if you haven't because you are concerned about their reactions, or they've been resistant to having these conversations, this chapter offers a few more tools.

As you work through these stories and exercises you will get a better idea of how all the pieces of advance care planning go together.

The importance of conversations:

- While 95 percent of people are willing or want to talk to loved ones about end-of-life, only 32 percent have done so.

- While 80 percent of people who are seriously ill want to talk to their doctors about their wishes for medical treatment, only 18 percent have had this conversation.

- While 97 percent of people say it's important to put their wishes in writing, only 37 percent have followed through.

(The Conversation Project, 2018: https://theconversationproject. org/wp-content/uploads/2017/02/ConversationProject-ConvoStarter Kit-English.pdf)

1. Talk to the People You Love

The hardest people to talk to about what we do and don't want if we are seriously ill or injured are our loved ones. You've been doing this work and you've had time to reflect on it — but it could be a shock for them. The thought of you being incapacitated or dying, even if it might be years from now, is often overwhelming.

Remember that you are giving them a gift by talking about this now. It can take the darker emotions — fear, anger, regret, shame — out of the shadows where you can look at them and talk about them. It may allow for healing and a less complicated grief for them when you die.

My father's path toward death was very typical: He had a major heart attack at age 72 and major open-heart surgery shortly after that. Then he had a series of strokes and infections that slowly took away his strength. He had not been an easy man to live with and there were as many bad memories as good ones. The gift he gave me was talking openly about the end of his life and how he wanted to die. We began to have deeper conversations. He talked about his upbringing and why he raised us with a heavy hand and so much anger. He apologized and I forgave him. His last few years were some of the best we ever had.

Having the first conversation with my own adult children about what I want —and don't want —if I am seriously injured or ill wasn't easy. But, once we had the conversation, I felt like I could take a deeper breath because if anything happened, they would know what to do and what to say. My daughter still groans when I bring something up that's important to me, but the conversations are easier every time.

Every person and every family is different. Sometimes wounds are too deep to heal and sometimes the thought of your passing may be just too big to handle. But trying to have the conversations is a good place to start. If you feel your family would benefit from mediation and reconciliation, consider local therapy and counselling services.

If you don't know how to start the conversation, write it out, and then ask your loved ones to allow you to read it to them.

Gloria had three adult children and five grandchildren. She was intelligent and feisty and the centre of her family. She had three separate bouts of cancer over the years and every time had found her way back to health, except this time. This time she was told that the cancer had spread, and it wasn't curable. She still looked the picture of health, but she didn't want to put off the conversation about her end-of-life wishes with her family any longer. She knew her children would be devastated, and then they would tell her to not give up – and they would want to look for alternative treatments. They would want her to fight.

She wrote out her values and beliefs. She said the quality of her last months was more important than spending them getting treatments that would buy her a few more months, at best. She wrote out that she wanted to go on a few more memory-making trips and, when her health began to fail, that she would like to die at hospice with her family at her side.

One evening, she asked her adult children to come to her home. She made tea and had their favourite cookies. And then she read what she had written word-for-word. Everyone cried, as predicted. But by reading out her values and beliefs, they understood what was important to her. The questions started to flow and then the conversations. I was there. It was an incredible evening.

1.1 A few ways to start your script

- I've been reading a book (watched a documentary; went to a workshop) and it got me thinking about what I would want for my health care and the end of my life if I couldn't speak for myself or make my own decisions. I know it might be a tough conversation but I'd like to talk about what's important to me.

- I know this is going to sound way too early in our lives to have this conversation but I'd like to start to talk about what we would want for ourselves if we are seriously injured or ill.

- I want you to know there is nothing wrong with me right now. With that said, there are things that are important to me if I'm seriously injured or ill, or if I develop dementia.

- What I need to talk to you about is not easy but it's really important to me that we take a few minutes to talk about.

- I'm going to need to depend on you to be my voice if I can no longer speak for myself. Sometimes we don't think the same way about things and it's important for you to know why I feel the way I do.

- My treatments aren't going well. I know it's really tough to talk about this but it's important to me that we do.

Include in your script:

- I value,

- I believe,

- I fear ...

- I would like the end of my life to look like ...

A few suggestions about what to say:

Write out what you want to say and practice it a few times. Try to stay logical because it can be a very emotional topic. If possible, practice with a friend.

What's important at the end of my life ...

When you are still well and healthy you can write:

- I want to talk to you about the decisions you may have to make on my behalf if I am very ill, or have dementia, and I can't speak for myself. Don't be concerned. There is nothing wrong with me. I'm just being proactive in talking to you about it. At this point, if I were to be seriously ill or injured, I want everything done. But, if things go sideways, I wanted you to know what I do and don't want in the way of health-care treatments.

- I was reading a book that got me thinking and I want to talk to you about what I would want if I were seriously ill.

- I'm getting older and I've been thinking about what I want done if I have a health crisis. I know this is uncomfortable but I really need you to listen and hear what I want and don't want if things are looking serious for me and you need to make some decisions.

It's often the toughest to have these conversations when we've received a life-threatening or life-ending diagnosis. You may have been told, "Come on, you've got to keep fighting this." Or, "You can't give up hope." There can vehement denial that you will ever die, let alone in the foreseeable future.

The perceived loss of hope gets in the way of heart-felt and necessary conversations and it's important to understand this massive four-letter word. Focused hope is based on doing; it is outward, tangible goals. Intrinsic hope is something we are all born with and allows us to focus on the goals of recovery and the discomfort treatments will cause. And, as our disease progresses, it allows us to focus on personal issues and receive love from family and friends. (The duel nature of hope at the end of life: The BMJ Opinion, April 2017.)

The thought of losing hope can shut down conversations. Switching the focus can make discussions easier: "I know that the doctors are telling us we're out of treatment options and that's devastating. I know this is really tough but I'm ready to shift my focus to having really good, quality of life with you and our family."

1.2 When you are speaking to your loved ones

When you are speaking with loved ones keep in mind:

- Be patient. Some people may just take more time to think.

- You don't have to steer the conversation. Just let it happen.

- Don't judge. A "good" death means different things to different people.

- Nothing is set in stone. You and your loved ones can always change your minds as circumstances change.

- Every attempt at the conversation is valuable.

- This is the first of many conversations — you don't have to cover everyone or everything right now.

2. When We Are Old and Frail: Conversations When We Are Coming to the End of Our Natural Lives

Conversations get even harder as we get older. Far too many older, frail adults spend their last days in critical care units, on ventilators and full life support because they have not thought about their wishes for future health care or have not discussed their wishes with loved ones and their doctors.

Thirty percent of frail nursing home residents are admitted to an intensive care unit and 50 percent to hospitals in the last year of their lives (Living Well, Planning Well, An Advance Care Planning Resource for Lawyers: Speak Up (Canada) December 2019: https://www.advancecareplanning.ca/resource/living-well-planning-well-lawyers-resource/).

As we age, illness, frailty, and end-of-life often creep up on us. For most of us, there is not a big diagnosis of cancer or a heart attack. It's often just old parts, slowly breaking down. The medical system keeps fixing those parts because there is no clear line of where or when to call it a day and let take nature take its course. These ongoing treatments are called "mission creep" and they can happen even if you have clear medical orders that call for no resuscitation or critical care interventions.

"Painful, futile treatment continues to this day, particularly with elderly patients who often are not informed of the difference between palliative care, designed to minimize pain while trying to preserve quality of life at the end, and aggressive treatment more designed to prolong life at any cost, using such methods as surgery or chemotherapy. Often, they are not informed about the benefits of letting some conditions run their course.

"Here in [North] America, there is a deeply held belief that advances in medicine will eventually conquer or cure the chronic scourges of cancer, dementia, heart disease, lung disease and diabetes. This notion leads many elderly patients to seek aggressive treatment not only to spare their loved one's grief but because they hope (and expect) to be cured, if only they hold on just a little longer." "Mission creep doesn't benefit patients at end of life," *The Washington Post*, August 2016.

Our loved ones are often our champions and cheerleaders as this creep continues on. I remember my father saying many times over the last few of his 91 years, "I'm tired. I'm done." My mom said, over and over, "Come on, Tom. It's just been a tough day (week or month). You'll feel better soon." Out of ear shot she would say to me, "He's just a little depressed. He'll be fine." She was his caregiver, cheerleader, and champion and he likely would have died 20 years before, if not for her. But it was a role that she simply couldn't let go of, even when she knew he had passed his "best-before" date, when every day was a chore, and he was no longer enjoying life.

Over the last ten years of his life he'd had a quadruple bypass and two valve replacements; five strokes, all relatively minor, but they had added up; but the simplest issue was the worst — and would eventually cause his death — bladder infections (also known as UTIs or urinary tract infections) caused by the superbug MRSA. Each time he would recover to a large extent, but it took longer, and his health baseline was never as high as before the most recent illness. The last two years of his life were a series of longer and more frequent hospitalizations that left both of my parents worn out.

I often wondered what we could have done differently — and when — as the medical creep kept along its path. If I knew then, what I know now, I would have sat down with him privately, and delved a lot deeper into when he said he was worn out and done. "What does that mean for you, Dad? You have choices. When you get another active bladder infection, do you want to leave it untreated? If something else happens — another heart attack or stroke — do you just want the doctors to leave you alone? Would you want to die, here at home, or do you want to go to the hospital?" And only after I'd had these discussions with him, would I have called in my mom, to have her truly hear what he'd said. We would have made a plan.

Listen to your ill or elderly loved ones. When they express concerns about continuing treatments, use it as an opportunity to open the conversation, and ask what they do and don't want for healthcare — such as antibiotics or resuscitation — and help them make their plans and documentation.

3. Talk to Your Physicians and Health-Care Providers

This shouldn't be the hard part. However, it often is. Doctors can intimidate us, and they know more than we do. They are by their nature and training, optimists and fixers. They don't want to show you they're giving up hope or dash your hope.

Eighty percent of Canadians think it's important to discuss advance care planning with a health-care provider but only 8 percent have, and Canadians say they would be more comfortable having ACP conversations if they had more support from health-care providers and other professionals ("Advance Care Planning in Canada: A Pan-Canadian Framework; Speak Up," Canadian Hospice Palliative Care Association, 2019).

Sam was 48 years old, was married, and had two teenaged children. He'd been diagnosed with a rare form of cancer two years before and had undergone multiple surgeries, three courses of antibiotics, and a round of radiation. Even though he had run out of options, he was reluctant to have a conversation with his doctors about his prognosis and end-of-life. As his weight continued to drop, as he had more and more serious health issues, he still said, "They're not telling me to put my affairs in order. I'm not going to be the one to bring it up." Sam died three months later without his doctors telling him the end was near and to get his affairs in order.

You're an empowered patient. You're the one who needs to bring up your concerns about your life and your prognosis. It's up to you to start these difficult conversations because your health-care professionals are waiting for you to bring it up.

When you book your appointment with your GP or your specialist, tell the medical office assistant that you want to talk about advance care planning and that you would appreciate some extra time. All provinces have a special billing code for these visits so you can get the time you need.

Like the conversations with your family, write up what you want to say to your doctors:

- Directly: "I want to talk about my wishes for end-of-life care."

- Bring in your written beliefs, values, and preferences and highlight the top ones that will be in your advance directive. Show the document to your physician. "I've written down my thoughts about end of life and would like you to see them."

- Share thoughts on someone else's death you have witnessed. "My father died a prolonged death from dementia, and I would want something different for myself."

Consider having your Substitute Decision Maker or a friend attend the appointment with you for emotional support, assistance in listening, and to reinforce their own understanding of your wishes.

If you have a serious or life-threatening diagnosis, ask the tough questions. Here are a few to start with:

- Will I need a specialist? When will I see him or her?
- Who is the doctor who will be leading my treatment team?
- What information will I need and where can I get it?
- What is my diagnosis and what stage am I at currently?
- Is my condition curable, chronic but manageable, or life-ending?
- What are the most important steps for me to take now?
- What do I tell friends, family, children, coworkers about my illness?
- Talk about pain control and symptom management options and let them know your preference between relief of pain or alertness.
- Share your thoughts on what is important to you; if you choose quality over quantity of life, let them know.

Give your doctor a copy of your completed directives and the contact information of your Substitute Decision Makers.

I really do know how tough these conversations are. I help people have them with their loved ones all the time; they can be emotional and draining for everyone. I procrastinated in having these discussions with my own adult children because we are taught not to talk about religion, politics, and death, but the consequences of not talking about it can be devastating and complicate grief.

The conversations must take place, one way or another —before you die, or afterward. You are giving all who love you a massive gift by having them now.

CHAPTER
TWELVE
Considerations for an
Empowered End of Life

Empowerment is informed choice. Informed choice at the end of life is what advance care planning is all about.

Every person's death is as unique as a snowflake, and it is utterly unpredictable. I have been with hundreds of people as they approached the end of their lives and as they died, and very few of them had a death that was as expected. Often, people don't die of the disease they were diagnosed with, but complications of that disease.

Some seemingly healthy people die between breaths (their bodies simply and suddenly stop) where others linger on for weeks after they quit eating and drinking.

Despite unpredictability, there are things you can do to plan, because planning often means a good death, or at least a better, more appropriate death.

What is a good death? That's largely up to you and is based on your values and beliefs. Most of us would choose to die at home (but few of us do). Nearly all of us would not choose to be in pain, but there are some who would choose pain so they are fully aware of being engaged with their loved ones as long as possible. There are some who choose Medical Assistance in Dying (MAiD) so they die fully on their own terms, in their location of choice, by themselves, or with their loved ones.

What a good death means is as unique as you are.

No matter whether your death is from serious illness, is a slow decline, or a sudden death, a good death is knowing that you have attended to all that you could, that you've talked to your loved ones and your decision makers about what you want and don't want at the end of your life, and where you can, you've put your choices and thoughts down in writing. If the people around you know what is important to you, they can honour you and your wishes.

In Canada, we have some of the most robust laws in the world about patient choice and how you can choose the way you want that to look. It is your choice to raise your voice and enact those rights.

Rights are one thing but access to care is quite another. Unfortunately, there are many gaps in health-care funding, particularly around the availability of home care, palliative, and hospice care that can hamper your ability to access the care you need in a location you that is close to home and family. That doesn't mean we shouldn't try to get what we are entitled to; it just means we must be more informed and more assertive. This is where the squeaky wheel gets the grease.

When the information is coming at you fast or relentlessly, you have a right to ask for a pause, to gather information, and the right to withdraw treatment.

Our health-care system can roll right over top of us and then drag us along, whether we want to go along for the ride or not.

When you have been given a life-threatening or life-ending diagnosis it is up to you to say, "Stop, I need to take a moment. I need more information. I need to listen to myself and what is best for me (or my loved one)."

Except in the most dire emergencies, you have a choice. Always.

Such was the case with my patient, Ed. I'd been a cardiac nurse for years and I knew that doctors often give patients little information and less choice. Ed was 85 years old and had critical coronary artery disease — he had several heart vessels that had greater than 80 percent blockage and the risk of sudden death was high. He had angina (chest pain due to lack of oxygen to the heart) with any exertion. His quality of life was not great but he had a lot to live for: He and his wife would be celebrating their 50th wedding anniversary in two months and their first great-grandchild was coming into the world a month after that.

I was with the cardiac surgeon when he came to see Ed. He said, "I've looked at your heart catheterization images and your heart is not in great shape. Chances are pretty high that without open heart surgery you could die at any time. There really isn't any choice: You need to have an emergency quadruple bypass. What would you like to do?"

Ed looked like a dear in the headlights. "If you say there isn't any choice, Doc, then there isn't any choice. Let's get it done."

"No, " I wanted to say. "Take a moment. Ask some questions. Ask for your wife and adult children to meet with the surgeon. Ask, Can I say, no? Can I go home and spend my last days with my family instead of here? I've got diabetes — is that a risk factor for surgery and what would that mean to my recovery? At my age, do I have a bigger risk of complications? What are those complications? Yes, I'll have a risk of sudden cardiac death but that's not such a bad way to die."

The cardiac surgeon didn't bring up value of the surgery versus risk and complications, or chance of dying on the operating room table or of post-operative complications. What he said was, "Good. I've scheduled for emergency surgery this afternoon. I'll get Connie to bring in the consent form and get you ready to head to the OR."

I let the doctor leave the room and I sat with Ed and asked if he had any questions and if he'd like to call his wife and kids. "There is always choice," I said to him.

He said, "If the surgeon says this is the only choice, then this is the only choice. I'll let my family know I'm on the way into surgery." He gave away his power and his right to choose.

Maybe, even if he'd asked all the important questions, he would have still proceeded with the surgery. But it would have been more informed and that is always a good thing. In my experience, patients who have asked for and been given more information react better and are more at peace with the outcome, no matter what it is. When they have not been given the important information, they tend to be much angrier when the outcome is not optimal.

The number one question of the empowered patient or caregiver is "What are the risks of the surgery (or treatment) versus its value?" No one has crystal balls. Some patients in their 80s do extremely well after open heart surgery. But, with more risk — things like diabetes, prolonged use of steroids, mild to moderate kidney failure, inadequate nutrition, frailty — the chances of going home without complications start to drop.

Ed did very poorly during the surgery and was in the cardiac surgery intensive care unit for more than a week. When he came back to the nursing unit, he developed an infection in his sternum (the broad chest bone that is cut during surgery and then put back together with wire) which is more common in diabetics. He was with us for six months and he died in the hospital.

If he had said no to the surgery — after taking a moment to ask questions and consult with his family — he might have gone home instead. He might have had his anniversary while sitting in his reclining chair and oxygen on with his family gathered around him. He might have held that first great-grandchild in his arms. He could have died at home.

You're allowed to say, "I need more information." You're allowed to say, "It's time to stop." You're allowed to say, "No."

Saying any of these things does not mean you are giving up hope. Your version of hope just shifts and it is based on your values and beliefs, such as:

- I believe in quality of life over quantity.

- If possible, I want my last days to be at home, with those I love.

- I want to go and make some memories with my family rather than try one more (treatment, drug trial, surgery).

- Yes, I want this (treatment, drug trial, surgery) but I want to re-evaluate before moving forward again.

1. Choice When Approaching a Natural End of Life

There are many serious, life-threatening, and life-ending illnesses with a slow downward trajectory: congestive heart failure, chronic forms of cancer, chronic respiratory disease, diabetes and its complications, neurological diseases, and end-stage kidney failure — but the biggest is old-age and frailty: "A fatal chronic condition in which all of the body's systems have little reserve and small upsets cause cascading health problems." (Living Well at the End of Life: Adapting Health Care to Serious Chronic Illness in Old Age: Rand.org: www.rand. org/content/dam/rand/pubs/white_papers/2005/WP137.pdf)

Decisions ending with "Enough is enough. I'm ready to die now," are difficult. It is where what-ifs come into play. Where am I on this trajectory? What if you give me one more round of antibiotics? What if we try a short trial on a ventilator? What if he rallies like last time? What if her heart stops but you can restart it?

This is where the hard conversations with doctors are necessary. What would it look like if we sent dad back to hospital if he gets pneumonia? What are his chances of not only surviving but thriving? When is it okay to say, let's stop: no more antibiotics; no more dialysis; no more feeding?

Talk to your doctor and ask for an honest, compassionate discussion about your values, beliefs, and preferences for care at the end of your life.

2. Choice at End of Life

We've been hiding death behind a curtain for a long time now. We've pushed back the timeline and death has come later and later. But death is inevitable. And there are many people who are pulling back the curtain and looking at it head on.

There are hundreds of people I know who are helping patients and families through their end-of-life journeys. We talk about death openly. We climb into caskets, and practice draping bodies. We look at the latest and most creative options for cremation urns. I feel more alive when I am with these people than when I am in any hospital or intensive care unit, where death is still hidden behind curtains and hushed into silence.

We want a little bit of the way things used to be back in people's lives: death at home, surrounded by loved ones, rituals and ceremony, celebration, and open grieving. More and more people are taking their deaths back into their own hands and making brave and beautiful decisions.

3. End-of-Life Options

3.1 Palliative care and hospice

All of hospice is palliative care, but not all palliative care is hospice.

Palliative care, and the medical subspecialty, palliative medicine, is specialized medical care for people living with any serious life-threatening or life-limiting illness. Palliative care is most often associated with cancer but it also includes heart disease, stroke, Alzheimer's, Parkinson's, and other neurological disorders such as ALS and Huntington's, kidney disease, diabetes, dementia, and other serious illnesses. People can receive palliative care for weeks, months, or years.

Palliative care focuses on providing relief from the symptoms and stress of living with a serious illness with the goal of improving the patient's quality of life for the time that is left, and sometimes, that is many years. It includes physical care, and psychological, social, and spiritual support.

Hospice care is provided as death approaches, and home or facility services are often offered in the last weeks or months of life. Hospice services also provide support for loved ones during and after death.

People who have access to and receive home palliative and hospice support live longer and their symptoms are managed better. They are admitted to hospital less frequently and are more likely to die at home (Living Well, Planning Well: An Advance Care Planning Resource for lawyers — Canadian Hospice and Palliative Care Association: www.advancecareplanning.ca/resource/living-well-planning-well-lawyers-resource).

Despite the enormous advantages for receiving palliative and hospice care, these services are not constitutional rights for Canadians. Many adults who have life-threatening and life-limiting diagnosis are not offered these services early enough, if at all, and many more don't have access to these services. If you are interested in becoming an advocate for increased services for all Canadians, please consider calling your provincial palliative and hospice society, the Canadian Hospice and Palliative Care Association, and/or your MP and MLA.

At home or in the community, if you have a life-limiting or life-threatening diagnosis, call your local Home and Community Health Office for home palliative and hospice assessment and services. You do not need a doctor's referral to open a request for services.

In hospital, if you would like to discuss palliative and hospice care options for any reason, but especially if you have been told active treatment is no longer an option, or you are thinking of asking for active treatment to be withdrawn, ask to speak to the nurse in-charge, the social worker, or (in larger hospitals) the palliative care team.

See Resources on the downloadable forms kit for further information.

4. Medical Assistance in Dying (MAiD)

On June 17, 2016, following a landmark Supreme Court ruling, federal legislation of Bill C-14 was enacted, allowing adults to choose Medical Assistance in Dying — generally known as MAiD (Supreme Court of Canada Ruling: Medical Assistance in Dying (overview): www.justice.gc.ca/eng/cj-jp/ad-am/scc-csc.html, accessed March, 2020).

It is assisted death and is no longer called physician death, assisted suicide, or euthanasia.

There is no cost to have MAiD as long as the recipient is covered by provincial health plans.

Adults have the choice to have MAiD performed at home, in the hospital, or in a palliative or hospice care unit. (There are still some religious facilities that have opted out of having MAiD performed on-site. They must arrange for the adult to be transported to a facility that does support administration. This can be a hardship for adults who are at end of life and are already suffering.)

The practitioner will remain with the adult throughout the administration. Most of the time, the sedation and medications that cause death are administered by an intravenous (IV) route through a small plastic canula. The adult is first put into a deep sleep followed by the administration of medications that cause death. The whole procedure is done in minutes.

If an adult chooses to take the medication orally, a strong anti-nauseate is given first to reduce the likelihood of vomiting. Oral medications take more time to work and in most instances, the practitioner remains at the adult's side in case of vomiting, other side effects, or if it does not work effectively to administer the medications through an IV.

On February 24, 2020, the Ministry of Justice and Attorney General of Canada introduced a bill, which proposes changes to the Criminal Code's provisions on MAiD. Proposed changes to Canada's medical assistance in dying legislation: Government of Canada, Department of Justice: www.justice.gc.ca/eng/csj-sjc/pl/ad-am/index.html (accessed March, 2020).

Adults who are suffering greatly *but whose natural death is not reasonably foreseeable* (for example: those with severe, chronic pain or otherwise debilitating disease) would, if the changes are approved, be eligible for assessment for MAiD and can receive it, if they meet all other qualifications.

Adults who may lose mental capacity due to advancing disease conditions, or the need for medications that might diminish their ability to make decisions, will now be eligible for assessment for MAiD and can receive it, if they meet all other qualifications, even if they lose capacity. This is called an *Advance Request*.

The proposed changes are expected to receive ascension and legislation. It is an evolving area of law, so check government websites for the latest development.

4.1 When the people you love don't support your decision (or you don't support your loved one's decision)

Family opinion matters to most of us. And, it likely stops people from making the decision to have MAiD. But others move ahead with it, choosing not to involve those who are opposed. Others choose not to tell the people they love of their decision — and to never divulge their cause of death and to simply have the doctor say, "She died peacefully." Period.

If you can, try to talk openly with those you love about your decision to have MAiD. Let them know why you have chosen this option. This is a new concept for most of us and some will not go happily down this road with you. If you are facing opposition to your choice to have MAiD, reach out to therapists, counsellors, facility social workers, or Dying with Dignity Canada for support.

5. A Few Growing Professions and Options for Your Life's Ending

5.1 End-of-life doulas

End-of-life doulas are helping to transform the way our culture approaches the process of dying. They are "death coaches" and they are objective, non-family members who can help the dying and their loved ones to turn something to be feared into an event to be celebrated. They are end-of-life navigators who work with and enhance palliative and hospice services and provide support aligned with the person's beliefs and values. They can bring peace and a sense of closure.

Many EOL Doulas belong to the End-of-Life Doulas Association of Canada. Their mission is to raise the standard of End-of-Life Care (EOLC) and their vision is to set standards through membership and training based on need and recommendations made by the Ministry of Health, health authorities, and outside agencies such as Canadian Hospice and Palliative Care Association.

They are advocating for End-of-Life Care Doulas to be seen as a part of the palliative care team and advocate for more funding to be put into end-of-life care, so that regardless of finances, everyone will be eligible to receive a doula.

If you would like to learn more about becoming an EOL Doula, or if you would like to hire a doula, contact the EOL Doula Association at endoflifedoulaassociation.org.

5.2 Alternatives in death ceremony

The rules are gone when it comes to funerals. Death care is being rewritten. Independent cremation and funeral services are opening all over the country, offering compassionate choice and alternatives including green burial and unique ceremonies.

If you want to find an alternative funeral or cremation, here are some key-word searches for alternative cremation and burial services: [your city or area], death, cremations, funerals, green burial, ethical practices, greener alternatives, personal values, natural options, celebration, minimal environmental impact, death at home, home visits.

Download Kit

Please enter the URL you see in the box below into your computer web browser to access and download the kit.

www.self-counsel.com/updates/adcareplan/20kit.htm

The download kit includes:

- Checklists for hospital stays
- Worksheets from the book
- Resources for further reading